Gaza

A Doctor's Diary

Dr. Salman Khalid is an attending Emergency Physician with 15 years of clinical experience. His medical mission to Gaza was his first time practicing medicine in a conflict zone. He lives outside of Toronto with his wife and three children.

Gaza
A Doctor's Diary

Salman Khalid

Foreword by Fozia Alvi
Afterword by Diana Buttu

PLUTO PRESS

First published 2025 by Pluto Press
New Wing, Somerset House, Strand, London WC2R 1LA
and Pluto Press, Inc.
1930 Village Center Circle, 3-834, Las Vegas, NV 89134

www.plutobooks.com

British Library Cataloguing in Publication Data
A catalogue record for this book is available from the British
Library

ISBN 978 0 7453 5164 3   Paperback
ISBN 978 0 7453 5142 1   EPUB

This book is printed on paper suitable for recycling and made
from fully managed and sustained forest sources. Logging, pulping,
and manufacturing processes are expected to conform to the
environmental standards of the country of origin.

Typeset by Stanford DTP Services, Northampton, England

Simultaneously printed in the United Kingdom and United States
of America

EU GPSR Authorised Representative
LOGOS EUROPE, 9 rue Nicolas Poussin, 17000, LA
ROCHELLE, France
Email: Contact@logoseurope.eu

For my friends, colleagues, and patients in Gaza

Foreword

Dr. Fozia Alvi

عَلَى هَذِهِ الأَرْضِ مَا يَسْتَحِقُّ الْحَيَاةْ:

We have on this land that which makes life worth living
– Mahmoud Darwish, Palestinian Poet.

I vividly recall that July evening when I met Dr. Salman Khalid, an emergency medicine physician, in an introductory virtual meeting. He was meticulously chosen by our director from a distinguished pool of 38 physicians to join Humanity Auxilium's September 2024 medical relief mission to Gaza. Though it was my first interaction with Salman, the agitation in his voice, the anxious disquiet, and the overwhelming sense of urgency to help the people of Gaza mirrored my own spirit before I went to Gaza on February 11, 2024 and even at present. We found common ground in our collective misery, in the futility of the situation, and most of all, our powerlessness. Within the first few minutes, I resolved to send Salman—the resolute energy in his desperation brought back memories of my own first mission.

In 2017, I traveled to Cox's Bazaar, Bangladesh on my first medical mission to help the Rohingya refugees as they poured in from Myanmar. While providing medical aid to the survivors of a modern-day genocide, I came to the painful realization that my time there was far too short, and much more was needed. The desire to do more led to the establishment of a non-profit, international non-governmental organization, Humanity Auxilium. Since then, I have witnessed the suffering of countless individuals—from those fleeing conflict zones to those enduring the aftermath of natural disasters. Yet, nothing prepared me for the grim reality of Gaza.

As a family medicine physician, I am used to treating patients of all ages. However, I was unprepared for the heart-wrenching reality of encountering so many children—innocent lives shattered with shrapnel and bullet wounds. I witnessed a generation of amputees, children robbed of their childhood and broken in unmendable ways. I saw mothers consumed with grief, unsure of which of their children to mourn—the ones killed, the ones clinging to life, or the ones left broken, with limbs torn away. I went there to heal them, but I returned wounded in ways I hadn't anticipated.

This journal, written by Dr. Salman Khalid during his 29-day deployment to Gaza, stands as an unprecedented testament to the harrowing experience—no other physician has so thoroughly documented the personal and medical toll of this genocide. Reading Salman's journal brought the numbers to life, reminding me of the faces behind the figures. His firsthand account from the frontlines, treating the injured in Gaza's overwhelmed Al Aqsa Martyrs Hospital, paints a powerful picture of human suffering and courage without the barrage of images of trauma on social media that we consumed for months.

We have seen images of the carnage on our screens, and to some extent, are now desensitized. However, when we read about this same destruction in the journal, it resonates on a deeper level. It stirs a more profound agony within us—one that transcends the numbing effect of the images we've grown accustomed to witnessing, and makes the suffering feel all the more real and unbearable. While Salman originally wrote his journal to share privately with close friends and family, reading it revealed a profound truth—the world deserves to witness the raw, unfiltered reality of medicine practiced amidst genocide. Through Salman's lens, we see not just the medical crisis but the profound emotional and psychological toll borne by both patients and caregivers.

Salman's journal captures the distressing moments where medical staff, often overwhelmed and exhausted, must balance their own emotional strain while providing care to those whose suffering seems beyond comprehension. For patients, the anguish is not only in their wounds but in the loss of their loved ones, their homes, and an unlived life. For the caregivers, it is the constant battle to remain hopeful and compassionate in the face of abysmal despair, as they witness not only the brutality of the genocide but the long-term scars it leaves on the spirit. We also witness the remarkable resilience of the people, especially the local healthcare workers who continued to provide care while bearing the weight of grief and anxiety for their own family members—"Every time we come to work, we worry our family will be bombed. Every time we hear a bomb, we wonder if it hit our neighborhood or our home."

Salman shows us the silent battles fought in the corridors of Gaza's hospitals—the unspoken trauma of choosing who to save and the emotional fortitude required to keep moving forward with the guilt of not saving everyone. Yet, amid this pain, is an undeniable strength—an unwavering commitment to heal, to help, and to give whatever is possible to those in need. The many Khalils (a name that translates to "friends") we meet through Salman take us on a roller coaster of emotions ranging from pride for standing in solidarity with the people of Gaza to justified shame for existing in our own bubbles of safety as we return home.

As I write this foreword, the smiles, the tears, the stoic expressions replay in my mind like a haunting reel, and I am left to wonder how many of them have since faded away. I often find myself gazing at the World Health Organization dashboard for the occupied Palestinian territories, fixated on the ever-increasing toll of this genocide: 45,936 killed in Gaza, and an astonishing 109,274 reported injured as of January 8, 2025. I refuse to accept these figures as mere statistics; they represent real lives—each one with a past to celebrate, a present to mourn, and a future forever buried. These numbers fail to capture the full weight of the tragedy, the depth of the pain, or the extraordinary resilience that continues to shine through despite the devastation.

Through this journal, we come to realize that the crisis in Gaza is not only a test of human endurance and compassion, but also a call to amplify the silenced voices, shedding light on those whose stories have long been unheard. It is a reminder that the strength to find hope, even in the darkest of times, is rooted in the very essence of what makes *life worth living on this land.*

Dr. Fozia Alvi
President & CEO, Humanity Auxilium

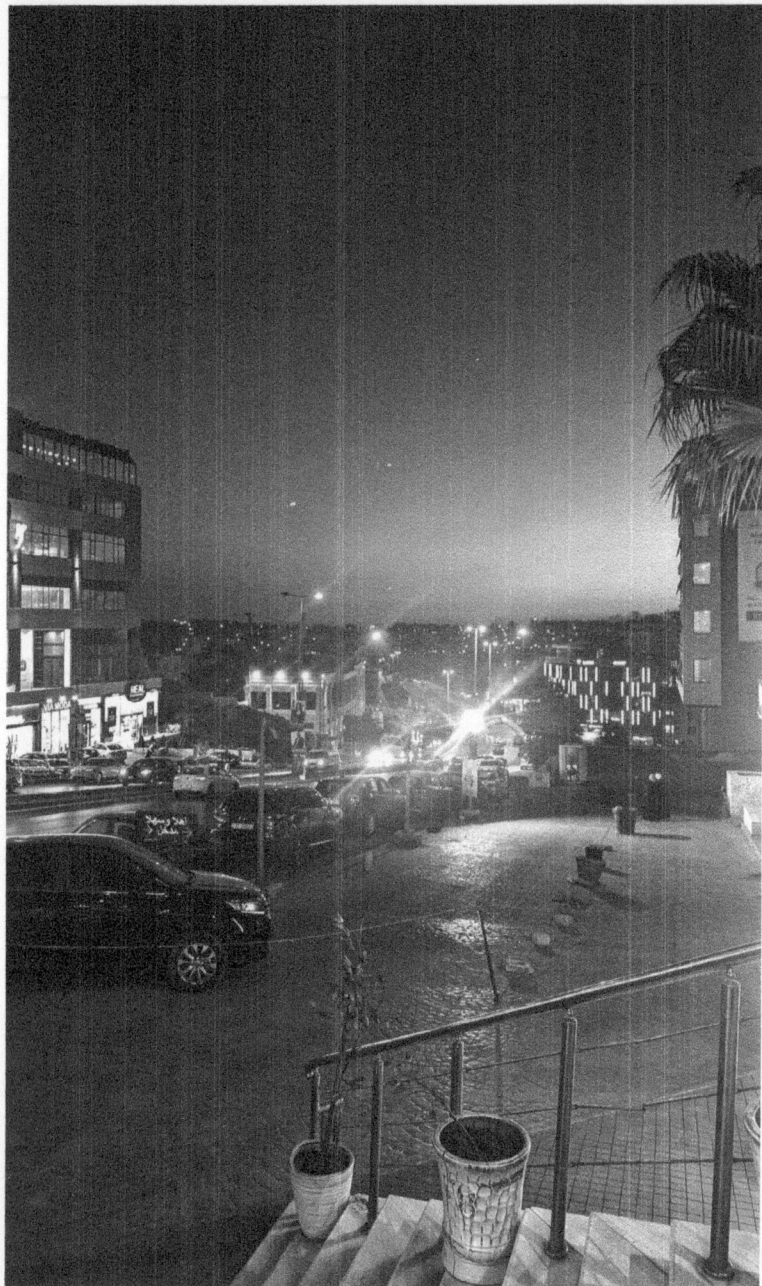

Night time in Amman, Jordan

Day 1
August 31 – Arrival in Amman

If you are reading this, then know that you are dear to me and/or that myself or someone you know believes you have the ability to inspire and motivate those around you.

My name is Salman Khalid and I am an Emergency Physician practicing in Canada. My wife of ten years is also an ER physician. We have three children: our eldest daughter is six years old, our middle son is four, and our baby girl (not so much a baby anymore) is two. I share these details to provide some background into who I am and to provide context to my motivation in undertaking this journey.

The first few posts in these reflections will unfortunately be selfish posts about myself and my mindset. But then, I hope to pivot my focus to the people I hope to serve beginning on September 3rd.

Today is August 31, 2024, and I have just arrived in Amman, Jordan, with the hopes of entering Gaza on September 3rd as part of a collaborative team involving the United Nations, World Health Organization and the non-governmental organization (NGO) Humanity Auxilium. I say "hope" because there is increasing uncertainty whether or not our team will be allowed access into Gaza. The humanitarian corridor appears to be narrowing daily, and it is still unclear which of the few remaining functional hospitals we might be assigned to. Regardless, our team is still scheduled to arrive in Amman this weekend and be fully prepared for our planned entry.

For those that know me well, I am a fairly private person who dislikes attention. I have Facebook as my only social media app and don't post about myself or family. This journey is an intensely personal one and by making these reflections public, I'm resisting my inclination to keep a low profile and maintain this as a mission to share only with my immediate family. However, this moment in time and our history is larger than my own feelings or preferences. As one of the lucky few foreigners to hopefully enter Gaza, I feel a sense of duty to the patients I will treat and the people I meet to tell their stories, especially in the absence of any foreign journalists. My primary role is to help serve the patients and medical staff who are exhausted and burnt out. The past eleven months have seen the near complete destruction of the hospital and medical infrastructure in Gaza.

For security reasons, we have been instructed to avoid posting anything on social media in real time, as it has the potential to compromise the safety of the medical personnel on the ground in Gaza.

I will do my best to maintain neutrality and avoid a political discussion. I will try to avoid using hyperbole and only report what I see with my own eyes. I promise to uphold the oath I took when I graduated from medical school 17 years ago, that all human life is sacred and worthy of compassion, mercy and healing.

In the past 48 hours up to and including my departure, I have experienced a wide range of emotions ranging from excitement and happiness, to anxiety, sadness and fear.

Much of my focus these past two weeks have been in preparing physically and emotionally for the journey, and also preparing our children for my departure. But I didn't realize how difficult it would be to say farewell to my family. It's a strange feeling: on the one hand, I can't wait to arrive in Gaza. But as I was saying farewell to my parents and siblings, and my wife's parents and siblings, I could see the worry and fear in their eyes. I know they believe in the importance of this mission but it was hard to escape the feeling of "this might be the last time I see you." I'm not a dramatic person and statistically speaking, I *should* be okay. But the past eleven months have seen the deaths of nearly a thousand medical workers, and more than 60 physicians. This is the highest number of any conflict in recent recorded history.

As an ER physician, I have seen many patients arrive in the ER who died in their sleep, and I truly believe that my time on this Earth has already been written for me. I am firm in my belief that I will be no closer to my death in Gaza than I would be in the comfort of my own home.

Despite this, saying goodbye to my three children was especially difficult. My four-year-old and two-year-old aren't aware of the gravity of my absence nor do they have a well-developed sense of what five weeks away means. They were still upset, but not like my eldest. She turns six years old in two weeks and knows full well where I'm headed, and the dangers that potentially await me. She's too young to understand and fully comprehend the reasons I need to be there. She only knows that my life is at risk and that she may never see me again, which still breaks my heart when I think about my kids growing up without their "baba." She knows

3

that doctors have been killed and that wearing a medical vest and stethoscope offers me no protection. She has been anxious and fearful since we first told her four weeks ago, thinking this would be enough time to allow her to process these emotions (and she has done an admirable job of it), but she has spent much of the past two days asking me not to leave. I simply have to accept (and hope) that she understands the meaning of this sacrifice when she is older, and is motivated to do the same when she is ready.

And my wife? What can I say about her? The first question that I am asked whenever I shared the news of my journey with anyone is "What does she think of this?" or "How is she feeling?" Everyone understands that it is largely through her selflessness and sacrifice that I am able to go. I can't even say she permitted this "reluctantly" or with any hesitation. My wife is a strong woman who has dedicated her career to the preservation of human life and dignity, especially for the most vulnerable among us. She is a woman of Yaqeen (certainty), who has felt the same pain and heartache over the past eleven months as I have. How fortunate am I that without me even asking, she would approach me in a moment of my own heartache and say, "I know you need to be there ... so go to them." She helped facilitate every part of this journey and linked me through her own contacts with Humanity Auxilium. I know her heart is also with the people and children of Gaza and she wishes she could be here with me, and I truly believe she will be rewarded as if we are here together.

The coming days will be filled with preparation and meetings with my arriving team members and briefings with the WHO and UN as we hopefully learn of our final destination in Gaza.

I hope you're willing to join me as I share this journey with you, and for you to share with others in the hopes that we can bring about a positive change in this world.

With love and respect to all my dear friends and family back home.

Your friend and brother, Salman

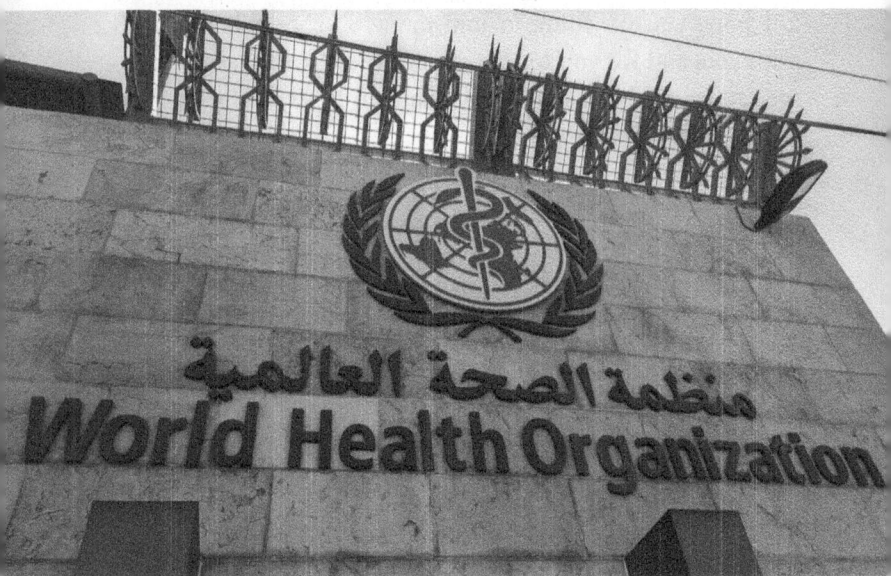

WHO Office in Amman, Jordan

Day 2
September 1 – Destination Confirmed

I tried to reset my sleep last night, but the combination of jet lag and nervous energy kept me awake from 02:00 to 07:00. I spent the time talking to family (Amman and Gaza are seven hours ahead of home) and praying, and ended up sleeping a few hours. I woke up at noon to attend a briefing, and meet my team members who arrived today. Today is also the day we learn which hospital we will be assigned to in Gaza.

The two other members of the Humanity Auxilium team are an emergency physician from the United Kingdom, Dr. Israar Ul Haq, and a general surgeon from New York, Dr. Victoria Aveson. Israar visited me in my room and greeted me with a hug like an old friend he hadn't seen in several years. I instantly felt a special bond with a person who has repeatedly left the comfort and safety of his home to serve in other humanitarian crises worldwide. He left his wife and four teenage children back home and this is his third mission to Gaza in 2024. Victoria arrived later and I met with her and was similarly awed by her previous global humanitarian work. The three of us met with Dr. Faiza Hussain, who is Humanity Auxilium's director of operations. She is based out of Houston and has flown to Cairo and now Amman to ensure our safe and prepared entry into Gaza, as well as to help coordinate the shipment of supplies into Gaza from their warehouse in Amman. The four of us had dinner together and spent the evening discussing and planning our coming weeks together.

By the end of our dinner around 8:00 pm, we finally received confirmation of the news that we had been eagerly anticipating for weeks: our entry into Gaza has been approved and we are assigned to Al Aqsa Martyrs Hospital in Deir Al Balah in Central Gaza where I believe we can be the most helpful.

Some background: Gaza is a strip of land measuring 40 km along the coast by 23 km. It can be divided into five regions from the northern border with Israel to the southern border with Egypt.

From north to south, these regions are North Gaza, Gaza City, Deir Al Balah, Khan Yunis and Rafah. Israel seized control of Rafah on May 6th and North Gaza and much of Gaza City has been abandoned by civilians since last October. What this means is that nearly the entire population of nearly 2 million people has been squeezed into an area of 40 square km (down from 360 square km last year), which is only double the size of Toronto International Airport.

These areas were designated humanitarian safe zones until two weeks ago when the Israeli Defense Forces (IDF) forced the population to evacuate these areas in order to perform airstrikes and a ground offensive. It was this most recent evacuation and ground operation that led to the uncertainty of whether we would be allowed access to these zones where we hoped our humanitarian work would take place. Just this past week, the United Nations evacuated hundreds of workers from the region and Al Aqsa Hospital was mostly abandoned for days. Fortunately, IDF ground troops have withdrawn two days ago, restoring the humanitarian corridor from which our team may now enter.

The recent ground operation has destroyed most of the homes in the region, so we expect the hospital to be sheltering many displaced families seeking refuge and medical care. I'm hopeful this means that the medical care we provide will focus around acute, chronic and neglected medical conditions, rather than the daily mass casualty incidents (MCIs) that have been the norm at Al Aqsa Hospital throughout August.

Tomorrow, we receive our final protocol briefing from the WHO and UN as we depart for Gaza in less than 36 hours.

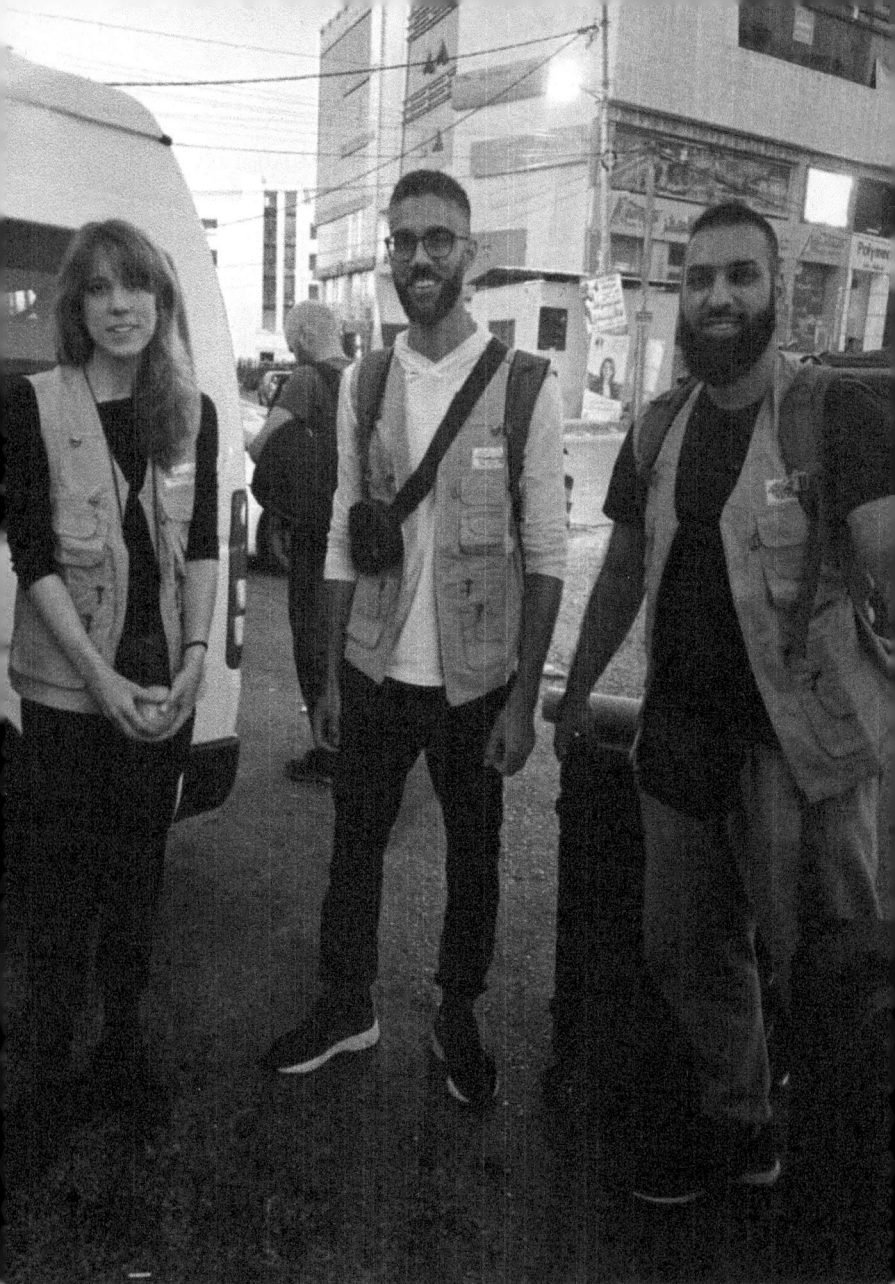

*Dr. Victoria Aveson (left), Dr. Salman Khalid (center),
and Dr. Israar Ul-Haq (right) prepare to depart for Gaza*

Day 3
September 2 – Anticipation

In the week prior to my departure, I began openly sharing my travel plans with my close friends. The second question everyone asked was "How can I help?" or "Can I send you money and/or supplies/medicine?" Due to the restrictions placed on the entry of humanitarian aid, including medicine and medical supplies over the past eleven months, it has been difficult to know which organization has actually been able to deliver aid directly to the people of Gaza. Having a friend enter Gaza removes this uncertainty and everyone I know has been keen to contribute. Unfortunately, there are enormous restrictions on what I may take with me now that the only entry point is through the Allenby Crossing from Jordan to Israel. The closing of the Rafah border in May has further worsened the delivery of aid into Gaza. Before Rafah closed, I was told of colleagues entering with over 20 suitcases of medical supplies. Because I'm entering from Jordan, I'm limited to a 50-pound suitcase and a 25-pound backpack of my own supplies (including most of my nutrition) required to sustain me for 30 days.

Also prior to the closing of Rafah, teams of between 20 to 30 individuals (emergency medical technicians, engineers, logistics) could enter Gaza every 7–10 days. Since May, the minimum length of a mission is now four weeks with the exception of a medical evacuation. Team sizes have also shrunk to 14 members allowed to enter weekly, and we are only allowed to take medical supplies for our own personal use. Any ideas I had of taking suitcases full of diabetes medications, insulin, antibiotics, etc. ended before they started. I'm also only allowed to take a maximum of US$2800. Trying to sneak in any extra funds will jeopardize the mission and the entire team will likely be turned away at the border.

The essentials that I packed are: 10 pairs of scrubs which I intend to wear and then give away, 28 protein bars, a laptop, 2 power banks, a LifeStraw bottle and straw to prevent waterborne diseases such as typhoid, cholera, giardia, dysentery and *E. coli*. I'm also carrying a personal trauma kit in my backpack, in the event I suffer an injury. This includes a chest seal for a penetrating chest injury, hemostasis gauze for a severe bleed, a metal tourniquet for an arterial bleed in an extremity, and a SAM splint for a broken bone (a lightweight, flexible and reusable orthopedic device). I'm allowed to take two phones in, and I've also packed 200 gloves and 100 masks. Six hours before my departure, I learned that the handheld Butterfly IQ portable ultrasound probe gifted to me by a friend will not be allowed in. This feels like a serious blow to my ability to deliver care, but I have no choice but to adapt.

Our team has now received requests from the hospital staff inside Gaza to bring cigarettes. The IDF allows each team member to pack one carton of cigarettes. I told our director of operations yesterday that I would need some time to think about the ethics of this request. I was leaning towards refusing until a conversation with Victoria (a cancer surgeon back in her home country) changed my mind when she said, "It's not going to be cancer that kills these people."

The second request our team received was for hospital scrubs. Many of the hospital staff where we are headed continue to work in old blood-stained scrubs and they were requesting clean ones. A search of Google Maps led us to a small shop. The store owner appeared particularly perplexed by my request for XL scrubs, trying to convince me that I would look terrible in them (my wife would have probably argued that they would have still looked better than my 14-year-old hospital issued scrubs that I currently wear to work). Eventually, we shared that we were taking these scrubs into Gaza. In an instant, his face changed and he became emotional. Speaking in Arabic, he expressed that he had been hoping and praying for months that he could send supplies into Gaza, and that the four of us walking into his store was the answer to his prayers. This man refused to accept payment and attempted to give us nearly everything in his modest shop. And I mean EVERYTHING. He refused to let us leave until he showed us everything we could potentially gift to a hospital in Gaza. Only when we explained our restrictions on medical supplies did he finally stop. We took his phone number and promised to direct future teams to him.

To top it all off, he limped across the street using his cane while we waited for our Careem (Jordanian Uber) to bring us water from a nearby shop. This wasn't an old man. He is in his mid-30s and had recently suffered a serious injury with multiple chest and pelvic fractures that rendered him bed-bound and unable to work for four months. He has only recently returned to work and yet he STILL refused to take anything from us except for what Israar forced into his hand. And then he used this money to try to pay for our ride back!

My three days in Amman have made me realize just how deeply the Jordanian people love the Palestinians. Nearly everyone we've met has said they would trade places with us in a second. We've even received requests to bring the *turaab* (earth) of Gaza back to people upon our hopeful return in Amman in October.

We had our final mandatory security protocol meeting with the WHO today and there was a lot to process. It felt as though every sentence ended with "but obviously anything can happen" or "as we all know, mistakes have happened."

September 3rd is the day that I have been thinking about every day for the past month. It is also the day that I have been the most nervous about. It is about a 10–14-hour journey by bus and car from Amman to Gaza, due to multiple vehicle transfers and military checkpoints. Once we pass the Karem Abu Salem Crossing from Israel into Gaza, we will be exposed to missile and artillery fire during our 2–3-hour drive in a UN-marked armored vehicle to our hospital. Our route will be "deconflicted" and we will be in the humanitarian zone, but this offers me little comfort as this was also the case with the World Central Kitchen workers and even ANERA last week. I don't feel like writing about it right now, but I encourage you to look up these events.

I simply have to accept that once I enter that vehicle (and even in this moment) nothing is under my control. Once I depart and start tomorrow's journey, I will be steadfast that my *du'a* (prayers) and those of my family and friends will be answered and I will pass safely into Gaza.

It is now past 1 am and our team departs in four hours. I need to sleep, but I doubt I will.

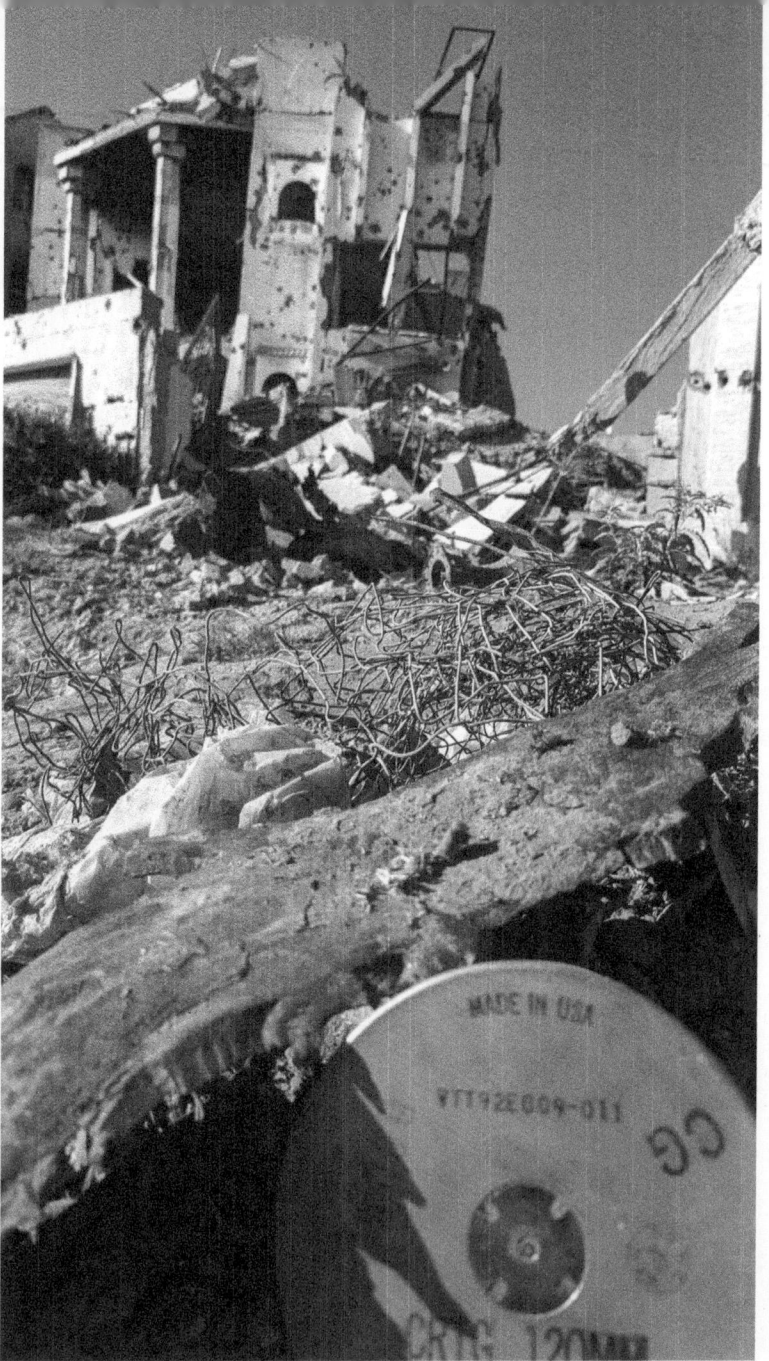

One of several mortar shells we found among the rubble in Gaza

Day 4
September 3 – Gaza

I'll get right to the point and avoid any suspense. Alhamdulillah, all praise to God, we have safely arrived at our assigned hospital in Gaza. It was a twelve-hour trip, involving two buses and two cars, and was uneventful other than the expected delays and secondary screening for no reason at the Allenby Crossing.

Let's start today at the Karem Abu Salem Checkpoint. Pictures are not allowed at this checkpoint from Israel into Gaza, but it isn't what I had imagined. It is a MASSIVE fortress-like complex spread out over miles with maze-like concrete walls rising 30 ft high (the same walls that surround the entirety of non-coastal Gaza). Our seven-vehicle armored UN convoy would drive from holding area to holding area. It was also here that the convoy donned Personal Protective Equipment (PPE), similar to the PPE that we use in the hospital. The only difference was that this PPE was Kevlar vests and bulletproof helmets. This was also the first time I heard the earth-shaking sounds of artillery and mortar fire from approximately 300–400 m away. The sound of each "boom" didn't bother or threaten me as they seemed distant enough to not cause us harm. But as a medical professional, what bothered me was the silence after each mortar fire as I imagined the human toll that lay at the landing spots.

Our convoy from Karem Abu Salem into Gaza con-
sisted of seven armored UN cars. Each car contained two
to three members of a separate humanitarian team from
organizations such as MSF, UNICEF, Project Hope and a
UN driver. The rendezvous point from where each hospital
would pick up their assigned team was a one-hour drive at
a speed of 10–15 km per hour along bumpy, makeshift dirt
roads. It was during this drive that the bleak reality of 2024
Gaza revealed itself.

At the very instant I was receiving pictures from my daughter's first day of grade one, our car was repeatedly swarmed
by tens of elementary school-aged children climbing onto
the roof and tapping on our windows asking us for any type
of help. I'm still shaken by our driver announcing "hard
brake in 3-2-1" and then jamming the brakes. I was totally
unprepared for how desperate children falling from the roof
of our car and onto the ground would affect me, and I still
can't remove the visual from my mind. We passed donkey
carts and a funeral procession, but most of all, we drove
by hundreds of barefoot, dust-covered children. Of the 2
million people in Gaza, half are children. Seeing all these
children wandering seemingly aimlessly through the streets
in search of the basics of life, I couldn't imagine a future for
them that was anything but desperate.

The second way in which Gaza revealed herself to us was
in the sheer scale of destruction and rubble. Once we passed
from Karem Abu Salem into Gaza, all one could see was
miles and miles of ash-colored, bullet-riddled, crumbled
buildings with exposed and twisted wrought iron wires. I
promised I wouldn't use hyperbole, so I'll need a few days
to articulate what I witnessed in a way that would do justice

to the destruction we were seeing. Despite watching all the television footage in the past year, the scale of destruction was incredibly disorienting to my senses. Our vehicle became noticeably somber as we slowly meandered our way through these streets. Our jovial British driver with over 30 years of experience in conflict zones stopped talking as well, as he also sensed the mood in the car changing. As if to validate that what I was seeing and feeling were real, I asked Victoria, "What are you thinking?" to which she replied, "I can't believe this is actually real. And how are there people still living here?"

On cue, her question was answered, as we drove by one of several large camps for the displaced. Calling them tent camps seems unfair, as they are more like random scattered places that were flattened and without rubble where a family erected a makeshift tent with sheets on a sidewalk less than 2 ft from the dirt road. Another aspect I was unprepared for was the overwhelming smell of raw sewage, as the sanitation infrastructure has been completely destroyed.

When we finally arrived at the rendezvous point, we met our handler for our trip, Dr. Muhammad Al Aqqad (aka Dr. Fowzi). He greeted us with an excited smile, along with his 16-year-old son and older brother at his side. We piled into his car and while driving he asked, "Would you like to see my home?" Our route was deconflicted and we didn't hear any drones overhead, so we took a risk and allowed him to drive us to his neighborhood. When we stopped the car we got out and followed him, hoping that he would show us something miraculous. As we got closer he pointed to yet another massive pile of broken concrete and twisted iron. "This was my home. My sister and her husband, and one of my brothers became "*Shaheed*" (martyred). People in Gaza use the term "*Shaheed*" to describe any of their loved ones who have died from the conflict. "It took me five years to build this house. I built it with my own hands" while his son showed me pictures of what his house used to look like. Then he smiled and laughed and said, "Alhamdulillah" (All Praise is due to God). "God willing, I will have a house in Paradise." He then paused and looked at us again and said with a steely-eyed resolve: "But don't worry, I'm going to rebuild it. Once this is over, I will rebuild it. And this will be the last one. I know this."

He then ran down the street to his other brother's demolished house where a date palm still stood. He picked off a handful of dates and shared them with us. Before Gaza was flattened, this man was a PhD lecturer at a local university which is now destroyed. And now he is living in a tent with his wife and five children. And yet, he STILL felt the need to feed us and host us from the ruins of his dream home. We would have stayed a few moments longer, but we could hear the drones getting closer and it was time to leave.

Just 30 minutes earlier, I drove by innocent children and saw only a bleak future. But this dignified man stood over the rubble of his home, remembered his dead loved ones and only showed *Shukr* (gratitude) and *Sabr* (patience) and not a hint of hate or anger. He stood on top of a pile of rubble, fed us and hosted us while dreaming and planning for a brighter future for him and his people. This is Gaza.

When we arrived at the hospital, we were shown the modest and comfortable room that Israar and I would share for the next four weeks, while Victoria was shown her separate room. The administration invited us to their boardroom and shared tea and dates with us as they welcomed us and introduced themselves. They then toured us around the hospital as part of our orientation.

When we arrived in the emergency department, my home for the next four weeks, it felt chaotic (even by ER standards) with hospital staff attempting to redirect distressed family members and perform crowd control. It turned out that our imagination at the sound of artillery at Karem Abu Salem came to life as a mass casualty incident (MCI) arrived at the ER one hour prior when a rocket or bomb landed on a house.

As we continued our tour towards the resuscitation rooms, we were introduced to a girl between 12 to 16 months old with multiple abrasions and charred skin. "She doesn't look terrible," I quietly thought to myself until the physician lifted the sheets to reveal an amputated left foot.

Resisting the urge to jump in and help, we continued our tour to the operating room, where we found the toddler's older sister being operated on. When we inquired about the child's injuries, the surgeon said she ruptured her small bowel and is currently having both legs amputated. Just two days ago, her parents vaccinated her against polio to protect her against becoming a paraplegic.

This … is … also Gaza.

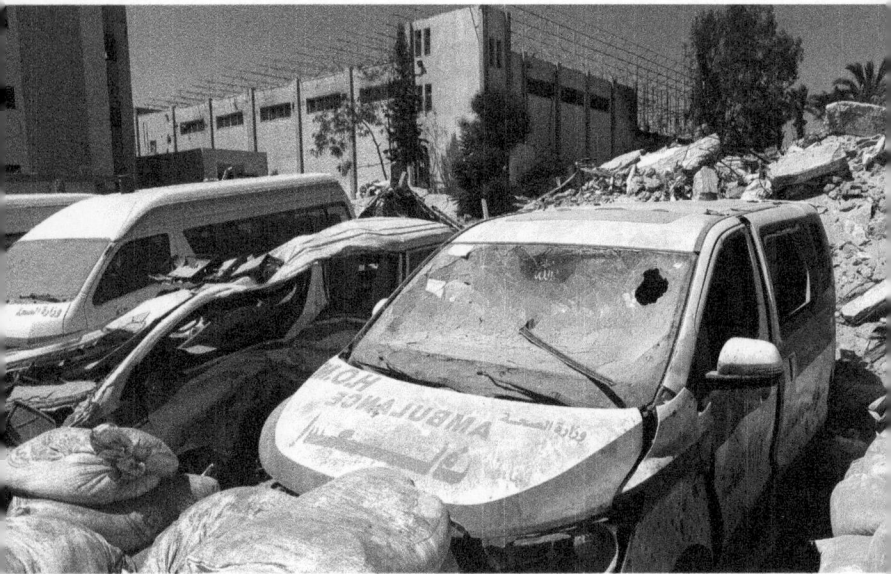

Destroyed Ambulances at Al Nasser Hospital in Khan Yunis

Day 5
September 4 – Getting Oriented

Our day began with a 10 am meeting with the Minister and Deputy Minister of Health in Gaza at Al Nasser Hospital in Khan Yunis. The two hospitals are only 18 km apart, but it took over one hour to arrive mainly because the streets were packed with people and it was difficult to navigate a vehicle around so much pedestrian traffic.

Our meeting included senior members of the Ministry of Health, and the administration of the remaining functioning hospitals in the region. This was an incredibly enlightening meeting where we discussed the current determinants of health in Gaza, including sanitation and sewage and access to clean water.

Nearly every determinant to health has been decimated over the past year, with the most visible being the loss of bed capacity due to the complete destruction of the majority of hospitals, and the loss of human resources due to the murder of healthcare workers. Despite a lively discussion on what global NGOs can offer to help rectify these issues, the ultimate solution is that the bombings absolutely need to stop.

A surreal moment came at the end of the discussion when these highly educated, brilliant and accomplished individuals broke out into laughter when talking about how they are all homeless and living in tents, to which I couldn't help blurting out "Wait, are you all actually laughing about being homeless???" They all simply said with good nature, "We are not happy, but we have no choice but to laugh." I have sat in hospital corporate boardrooms with senior leadership over the past five years, and all I could think was "how differently would the world act if it was our hospital leaders living in tents?"

We arrived back to our hospital at 1 pm and I tried to start work in the ER, but I quickly realized that I needed a more thorough orientation to the department. Israar was kind enough to take me under his wing and we spent some time learning the departmental flow and our access to resources.

The ER was even more chaotic and busy than yesterday, and we once again started in the resuscitation area, which is where most ER physicians gravitate to. The first patient we encountered was a 45-year-old male who fell from a height of 10 ft and had bilateral pneumothoraces with a suspected head injury and a positive FAST exam. In non-medical terms, he had collapsed lungs and bleeding in his brain, abdomen, and possibly chest. Tubes were inserted by the local doctors to both sides of his chest, and he was receiving a blood transfusion. In Canada, this patient would be rushed to receive a CT scan of his head, neck, chest, abdomen and pelvis, but our hospital CT scanner is broken, and they are not allowed to import the replacement parts to service it. He will have to be transferred to the hospital we visited in the morning to get this test.

The second patient we encountered was a four-year-old boy, who was the size of my two-year-old daughter. His home in the designated humanitarian safe zone was bombed today and he had a clearly visible depressed, occipital skull fracture. After waiting approximately 20 minutes, he was finally moved from his father's arms to a stretcher stained with what appeared to be fresh blood from the last patient and no mattress cover. While lying on the stretcher, his breathing became labored and he started decerebrate posturing (an involuntary extension of the limbs), which is a sign of a severe brain injury and impending brain death. He wasn't placed on oxygen or any cardiac monitor as the staff were just simply too overwhelmed with the high acuity in the department. He simply had no other option but to wait until he could be transferred to the other hospital for a CT of his brain and hope that a neurosurgeon can somehow intervene in time to save his brain and life.

I then moved to the tents outside the ER to see the non-trauma and medical zone. Here, I was introduced to a third-year ER resident, Khalil, as well as a staff ER physician, Anwar, who has completed his residency, but has been waiting the past year for a ceasefire and an opportunity to challenge his board certification exams. This is also an extremely busy zone of about 30 patients waiting to see a doctor, in a cramped 40x40-ft area. When I asked them which patients to prioritize assessing in this zone, they replied, "Whoever looks most desperate and grabs you by the hand first."

Before October of 2023, Gaza had 750 medical residents, doctors who have graduated from medical school and are performing an additional three to six years of training in a specialty (e.g. emergency medicine, cardiology, surgery, pediatrics, etc.). Today, that number has been reduced to 250. Some were able to escape, some have been killed, and many have had to leave their residency to support and travel

25

with their families after being repeatedly displaced. My heart aches for these young doctors. It was not too long ago that I was a resident and nearing the end of my training and dreaming of what my life and career would be like in the years ahead. I can't imagine how painful and unfair it must feel to have your career taken from you after several years of hard work and sacrifice to complete medical school.

Khalil helped me follow a 50-year-old male who presented to the ER with a cough, fever and weakness. He was clearly septic (which means there is bacteria growing in his bloodstream) just by looking at him and we diagnosed him with pneumonia, after performing a chest X-ray. The tragic aspect of this man's story is that he suffered a non-displaced hip fracture three months ago. He needed a surgery that never occurred or at least three months of bedrest. But due to the repeated forced displacements, he had no choice but to walk for miles on his broken hip. His X-ray today showed a completely displaced fracture with necrosis of the hip. If bombs continue to drop, this man will have no chance of getting the surgical treatment that will allow him even the hope of walking again.

I've now been in Gaza for 30 hours and away from home for five days. Everyone I have met has been incredibly warm and hospitable, and it is starting to bother me that I haven't really done anything useful for them since my arrival. I'm hoping I've got my feet wet enough to jump into work tomorrow and contribute in a meaningful way.

THERE ARE SILENCES
INSIDE YOU,
THAT YOU HAVE YET
TO EXPLORE.
THERE ARE THINGS
INSIDE YOU
THAT ARE STILL
FIGHTING A WAR.
SOME DAYS WILL BE
UNKIND.
SOME DAYS YOU WILL WANT
TO FORGET.
BUT STAY FOR THOSE DAYS
THAT ARE WORTH MORE
THAN ALL THE REST

Wars Inside You by Nikita Gill,
inscribed on the ICU Balcony at Al Aqsa Hospital

Day 6
September 5 – Losses

The explosion was a loud one. This one was close. At 4 am, an Apache helicopter fired three missiles into the tents inside the hospital grounds killing four people. It struck less than 100 m from where Israar and I slept. I made a promise that I wouldn't do anything risky or venture far from the hospital walls, but later in the day, I had to see the site with my own eyes. As mentioned in my first post, there are no foreign journalists in Gaza and I promised that I would tell the stories of the people here. I feel like events like this are often dismissed by people back home because there are only Palestinian journalists reporting them. My hope is that I've earned enough credibility in my professional and personal circles that I can be considered a reliable source of information.

The twenty destroyed tents were indeed inside the hospital grounds in what the IDF has marked as the safe humanitarian zone. Wearing our Humanity Auxilium NGO vests, Israar and I attracted a large group of people and children who wanted to share what happened. We saw the 4x4-ft crater with debris surrounding. The eyewitnesses surrounded us and told us the story of the traumatic experience and showed us the shrapnel designed to tear apart human flesh. Now, to be honest, I can't prove whether the four people killed were fighters or civilians. Their neighbors all believe they were civilians. The only thing I'm certain of is that all the people who gathered around us were clearly traumatized as this was not the first time that they rested their heads with their children and families for the night, in a place they were promised was safe, only to be woken by a terrifying, disorienting and horrific scene. We knew we had lingered long enough, as the crowd we attracted drew the attention of the drones overhead, so we hurried back inside the hospital.

Earlier in the morning, I finally got to meet the director of the ER, Dr. Fahd Haddad. I was extremely impressed with this man who is one of only two board-certified ER physicians at the hospital. He is the quintessential ER doctor in that he is a person of high energy and a short attention span, who can barely sit still for a moment. As we conversed in his office in the emergency department, he was constantly interrupted by patients with charts in their hand, requesting help. He didn't refuse a single patient or display any frustration with the constant interruptions, instead, choosing to patiently listen to them and order tests on their chart to reassure them that he would take care of them. He has 40 staff physicians on his roster, nearly all of whom are residents or volunteers. A volunteer is someone who has finished medical school, but has not yet started residency and is working shifts for free. The resident salary is approximately US$200 per month (a single piece of toilet paper is currently selling for US$8–10 in Gaza).

We joined him in the resuscitation room to discuss a patient, a 25-year-old male who ingested methanol two days ago in an apparent suicide attempt, and is now completely blind. Even though the damage had been done, he recommended the patient receive dialysis as there was still acid measurable in the blood. Dr. Haddad already knew what the patient needed without our opinion, but this was his way of welcoming us to his department and showing that he values us.

In the adjacent stretcher was a 17-year-old male with a history of congestive heart failure (CHF). His ejection fraction was 15 percent, which means that his heart could barely contract, and is by far one of the worst ejection fractions I've ever seen in a patient of any age, let alone a pediatric patient. He was sitting upright in a position called the tripod position, which is a sign of a severe respiratory distress. He appeared exhausted and nearing respiratory failure and cardiac arrest. This patient was taken to the Intensive Care Unit (ICU) for ionotropic support, which are powerful life support medications required to get his heart to squeeze. This kid is in the end stages of heart failure and needs a heart transplant that he likely will never receive.

After seeing a few patients in the medium acuity zone (Green Zone), we came back to the resuscitation area (Red Zone) to look after a 67-year-old male with urinary retention (unable to empty his bladder) and with worsening breathing. As time passed, he went into multi-organ failure and needed to go to the ICU. Israar and I spoke with the ICU physician who was sympathetic and agreed with our assessment and plan, but gently said, "Before last year, I would have taken him to the ICU but today I can't. I need to save room for the next mass casualty incident." We respectfully accepted his opinion and within one hour, this man was dead—a death that will not be counted in the official death toll because a bomb or bullet did not kill him.

Before we had a chance to move his body, the next MCI arrived. A bomb landed in a neighborhood tent community and we had three new patients: a 27-year-old man, his 30-year-old wife and their four-year-old son.

The husband suffered open fractures (exposed bone) of both of his legs with extreme soft tissue and bone loss, especially to his left shin, which did not appear to be completely attached to his ankle. He also had an open, compound fracture of his left arm. We couldn't even place him in a stretcher because there was no space, so he lay on a gurney on the floor while he shivered and was prepared for the operating room (OR).

His son suffered a shrapnel injury that pierced through his rectum and exited through his lower abdomen. He lay on his abdomen in agony on a stretcher on the floor while his bandages soaked with blood and pooled onto the floor. He also had to be rushed to the OR.

The wife and mother, named Faswad, was the final patient we tended to, not because she wasn't critical but because her injury was catastrophic. She lay on a sheet on the floor next to her husband with a large skull fracture that was leaking brain matter. She was still alive but taking sporadic deep breaths. She didn't die immediately, but rather spent an hour struggling and trying to take gurgling, deep breaths with frothy secretions that seemed to be choking her. There's a shortage of suction catheters, so the nurses reluctantly allowed me to use one after I pleaded with them. We held off on giving a dose of ketamine, as we didn't expect her to stay alive as long as she did, and mostly because there's very little ketamine left in the hospital. Eventually, we finally allowed her a single dose so she could die in peace. When she finally died on the floor in a pool of her brain and blood, the nurses moved quickly to move her from the floor to the morgue to make space for the next MCI.

I then decided to pass by the operating room to get an update on the father and son. The boy was stable and needed a colostomy due to his rectal injury. The surgeons repaired the father's right leg and left arm with external fixators, and repaired his left brachial artery which was spurting blood "like a fountain." They unfortunately had to amputate his left leg below the knee.

I found myself imagining how this man would feel when he wakes up to realize that he is missing a leg, his son will have to defecate in a bag for potentially his entire life, and his wife and mother of his child is dead. If I was in Canada, this shift would rank among the most difficult of my entire career, but it seems like this will be just another day in Gaza.

As I walked back to my room for the night, I passed by a group of children in the courtyard of the hospital (kids sheltering in the tents on hospital ground). They were playing a makeshift version of "Skip It" using a water bottle they filled with sand attached to a piece of rope. While watching them, I thought of a poem I noticed scrawled on the ledge of the ICU balcony where I went to catch a bit of the sunset earlier. I believe it's a well-known poem, but the words still resonated deeply after a long day.*

There are silences inside you that you have to explore.
There are things inside you that are still fighting a war.
Some days will be unkind,
Some days you will want to forget,
But stay for those days that are worth more than all the rest.

---

* Since my time in Gaza, I have learned the title and author of the poem: "Wars Inside You" by Nikita Gill.

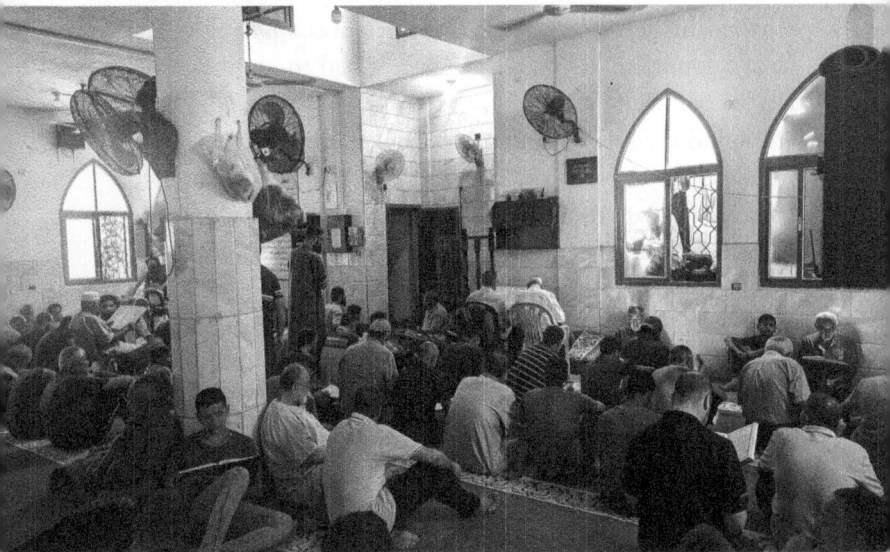

Friday Prayers at Al Aqsa Martyrs Mosque, in Deir Al Balah, Gaza
(October 6, seven days after our departure from Gaza,
this mosque was destroyed by a bomb, killing 26 worshippers.)

Day 7
September 6 – Jumah

One, three, seven … 13. Thirteen explosions between 04:30 and 05:30. These were all distant and didn't result in a mass casualty incident at our site. I'm starting to notice a trend of bombs exploding with regularity during the dawn hours, while people are either at home sleeping with their families or congregating for the dawn prayers. It's something that I need to keep track of.

The good from today: Israar and I spent four hours this evening resuscitating a 50-year-old man with mixed septic and cardiogenic shock (a severe infection, causing his heart to fail). The reason this felt like a win is that he received very near to the care he would have received during "normal" times in Gaza. The details of the case aren't as important as the idea that he appeared close to death when he arrived and four hours later, he was in the ICU and somewhat stabilized. There is still a greater than 50 percent chance that he will die, but the win comes from the idea that he was given the fairest and best chance at survival, which has not been the norm for the past year here in Gaza. This was also made possible by the fact that there was no mass casualty incident during the four hours we worked on him.

Today was also Friday (Jumah) prayers, which is the most important day of the week for Muslims. I built up the courage to attend with Israar and Dr. S (a Jordanian urologist from another NGO who has befriended and given me company in the late evenings, when I write my journal). The moment we were about to leave the hospital gates, their friend Mahmoud, a local Palestinian who lives in the neighborhood said to us. "Don't go, it's not safe." I immediately chickened out and told my friends: "Have fun fellas ... tell me how it was, and don't die" and went back inside the hospital. But as I made my way back inside, throngs of people were leaving the relative safety of the hospital grounds and tents to make their way to the mosque. Despite mosques being routinely bombed, including at times of congregational prayers, people were still walking across the street to fulfill their obligation. Mostly out of shame, I built up the nerve to again join the crowd and attend Jumah prayers.

When I ventured to write this journal, I did not have the agenda to talk about faith, and actually made the intention to avoid it altogether, making this solely about my experiences in the hospital and with the Palestinians. What I've come to learn in my first week here is that it is impossible to tell the story of the Palestinians in Gaza without talking about where they derive their strength and resilience. More importantly, it's the Palestinians themselves who have asked me to talk about their Islamic faith, and I owe it to them to tell their complete story, through their lens. There are also between 4000 and 5000 Christians still living in Gaza, but I likely won't be able to meet them and share their specific story, as their community is concentrated to an area I won't be able to visit.

I'm so grateful I attended Friday prayers because it allowed me to connect some dots. After a 20-minute sermon, the Imam of the mosque (the leader of the congregation) recited verses 153–156 from Chapter 2 of The Holy Quran. I encourage you to look up the meaning of these verses, which are the exact words I've heard every family member testify at the moment they receive the news of their loved one's death. Being present in this place, in this moment of history, standing shoulder to shoulder with these people and listening to those verses, I felt a calmness and sense of purpose I have never before experienced. It hasn't been all the tragedy I've witnessed thus far that has broken me but rather the patience and absolute submission they display in the worst moments of their lives that will cause me to weep long after I have departed from here.

After the sermon, Israar, Victoria and I were invited to Dr. S's room for lunch which was prepared by friend Mahmoud (the same Mahmoud who warned me against going to the mosque). He is 36 years old and lives in a tent nearby the hospital with his wife and children.

His wife prepared a traditional Palestinian dish called maqluba which is rice, chicken, fried vegetables and potatoes. We were also joined by our team's local handler Dr. Fowzi. Mahmoud and his family live in a tent nearby and are struggling with food insecurity like all Gazans, but they still shared their limited food supply with strangers and prepared a meal with love. The generosity and selflessness of the people of Gaza is something I hope I can embody upon my return home and instill in my children.

The bad from today: The first case of the day was a 17-year-old woman named Yusra, who suffered a catastrophic head injury with exposed brain from a bombing. She was brought to another hospital where they inserted a breathing tube, and I want to share this story for two reasons.

First, in Canada, when a patient requires a transfer to another hospital with more advanced services, the first hospital notifies the receiving hospital to discuss the case to ensure both sites are on the same page. In the past year in Gaza, there has been a complete breakdown in communication between hospitals, which means that patients like Yusra just show up at your door and you have to deal with them. Because of this, Yusra received a breathing tube that unnecessarily prolonged her suffering.

Second, the undignified way I've been watching people die is starting to affect me. Throughout my career, I've taken immense pride and spiritual satisfaction in providing end-of-life care to patients and their families in the ER who we can no longer offer or have failed life-saving treatments. Everyone deserves the chance to die in peace, comfort and surrounded by loved ones. Yusra (and most of the other deaths I've witnessed) spent the last hours of her life on the floor of the hospital covered in flies, with no immediate family present (because most have already been killed) in a pool of her blood and brain matter. The most attention she received was from the person who mopped her brain off the floor every 20 minutes.

No human being deserves to die like this, yet this is how most Palestinians have ended their life in the past year. I don't usually get emotional when patients die unless the patient is young or there is a unique aspect of their story that hits home on a personal level. But if I'm being completely honest, I'm finding myself getting increasingly upset with the lack of dignity, EVEN in death, afforded to the Palestinians living in Gaza. I am beginning to find it hard to find the words to begin to describe what I am feeling.

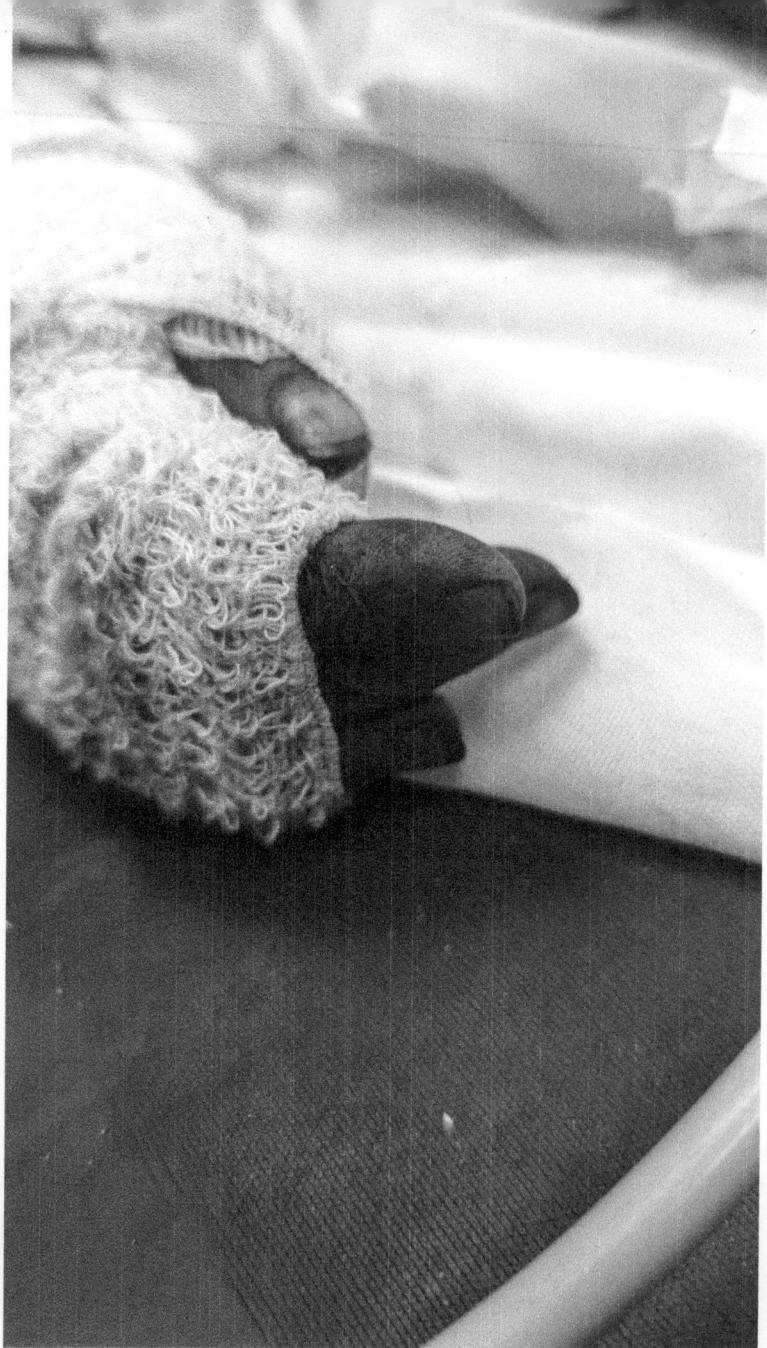

Misk

Day 8
September 7 – Kids

I didn't feel like writing today. I am tired. I am angry. I am questioning many of my core beliefs in the nature of human beings and what they are capable of. Today was the worst day. It was children. Only children. Suffering the worst atrocities of what some people are capable of inflicting. There can be no justification for this, right?? Or am I just naive and uninformed? Is it actually this "complicated"??

My day began as it usually does, with the sounds of explosions at 5 am. This time, the sound was followed by Apache helicopter fire. A loud rat-a-tat-tat … rat-a-tat-tat. That could have been just warning fire, or something much worse.

When we arrived at the ER in the morning, the chief of the ER, Dr. Haddad, was on shift and had just started reviving a nine-year-old boy with a blast injury to the head and chest. This was the longest resuscitation I have participated in since my arrival. After two hours, it became clear to Israar and I that this boy was not going to survive, so we looked at the leader of the code, Dr. Haddad, with the eyes that are familiar to any ER doctor. I've been on both the giving and receiving end of "that look" many times. My colleague would say "Salman …" followed by "the look" at the end of an emotional case that your heart doesn't want to give up on, but your brain knows it's time. It's only when your heart and brain align that the code leader has the courage to tell everyone "okay, stop" and declare a time of death.

Israar has known Dr. Haddad longer than I have, having been to Gaza on two previous humanitarian missions, so it fell on him to say the words, "Fahd, it's time" to which Dr. Haddad replied firmly, "No, we keep going. This is a special case. Let's readjust this tube and try again." His heart and brain hadn't aligned yet. A moment later, he shared why. This boy is the son of one of his ER nurses, and when we looked up, we realized that the father was at the foot of the bed wearing gloves. It all made sense now and we simply followed Dr. Haddad's lead, understanding he needed to keep going for his own closure. But once someone plants that seed of "it's over," it absolves the code leader of any imagined guilt once the death is finally declared. When everyone had stopped their efforts, Dr. Haddad whispered to Israar, "Okay, now I have to tell my friend that his son is dead." He walked over to the corner of the room where the boy's father was now standing and gave him a hug and whispered condolences in his ear. The father, although tearful, was calm and he continued to repeat "Alhamdulillah." Over the next 30 minutes, I witnessed many people visit their friend they affectionately referred to as "Abu Zayd" and offer their condolences. The boy's name was Muhammad Bassem and he was nine years old.

Anyone who spent time working in an emergency department knows the camaraderie you have with your colleagues, whether they be nurses, physicians, housekeeping staff, security, respiratory therapists, physician assistants, clerks, nurse practitioners or X-ray technician. It truly is a family. I can't even say a "second" family because you often spend more time with them than even your own family. You laugh together. You cry together. You celebrate some miraculous triumphs together and comfort each other when you feel like you failed. You fight with each other, and make up just as fast. You annoy each other. You miss important occasions on weekends and nights together. You do battle together and carry the scars together. You celebrate each other's happiest days (like weddings and the birth of children) as though they are your own, and mourn the sad days just the same. Most importantly, you love each other because outside of your immediate family, it's only your colleagues who truly understand the grind, and what drives you to do what you do.

So when Muhammad Bassem died, I felt like I knew how everyone felt. When Abu Zayd's colleagues hugged him, I knew the heaviness they felt. It hit home. But instead of having the chance to grieve together, they were robbed of these emotions as the two-year-old boy in the next stretcher, who had a chest injury from a bombing, began to crash. I thought this beautiful baby boy would be fine. He kept staring at me during the previous code and I even playfully ran my hand through his hair. I left the room to clear my head from Bassem's death and when I returned 40 minutes later, I was informed of his death. I wasn't even there to help.

I don't know if it's possible to rank what traumatic injuries are worse than others. But if I thought the worst part of the day was over, I was about to be harshly reminded in the worst possible way.

Two girls, age five and the other one six or seven. Another bomb, but instead of the usual crush injuries I've seen, they both suffered the full extent of the cruelty that these missiles/rockets/bombs were meant to inflict, shrapnel was embedded over their entire skin like tiny razor blades, all over their body.

And burns. Horrible burns. It doesn't do justice to describe them simply as second or third degree burns covering 40–50 percent of their total body surface area. These are horrific burns. Painful burns. Disfiguring burns. Soul-taking burns that left these young girls mutilated, with charred flesh that looked like it melted off their skin.

I'm not even close to being done describing this. The five-year-old had blood in her lungs and surrounding her heart, which meant that the shrapnel likely pierced her heart. She was rushed to the OR where she died. She had no family with her.

The six- or seven-year-old had left arm and leg injuries where the limbs were only attached by skin. In addition to her burns, she also had a catastrophic head injury. If all of this wasn't bad enough, her entire resuscitation took place on the floor. She was bandaged on the floor. Intubated while she lay on the floor. She was on the floor for hours. When she finally got a stretcher, Israar and I stood beside her, periodically swatting away flies and giving up after realizing it was a futile exercise. We reflected on how this girl reminded of us our own daughters—my eldest and his youngest. We watched her effortful breathing against the ventilator gradually slow until she passed away, which seemed like a mercy on her in some way. Her name was Misk—may her celestial scent match her beautiful name.

This journal was supposed to be therapeutic for me but I'm just as angry as I was at the start of this post, and now I'm just more exhausted.

When I shared my plans about this trip with people, several told me that what I'm doing is pointless and won't change anything. I know that they said this to try to talk me out of going somewhere unsafe, but maybe they were right.

In this moment, I'm reminded of the words of a colleague who was in Gaza in July, who wrote (paraphrasing): "at some point I transitioned from being a doctor to being a witness." That is what it feels like right now. I feel like all of my medical training and skills are essentially useless in undoing the carnage that I'm seeing. When I fail at that part, my only hope is that I can still keep at least half my promise, and tell their stories and be a witness.

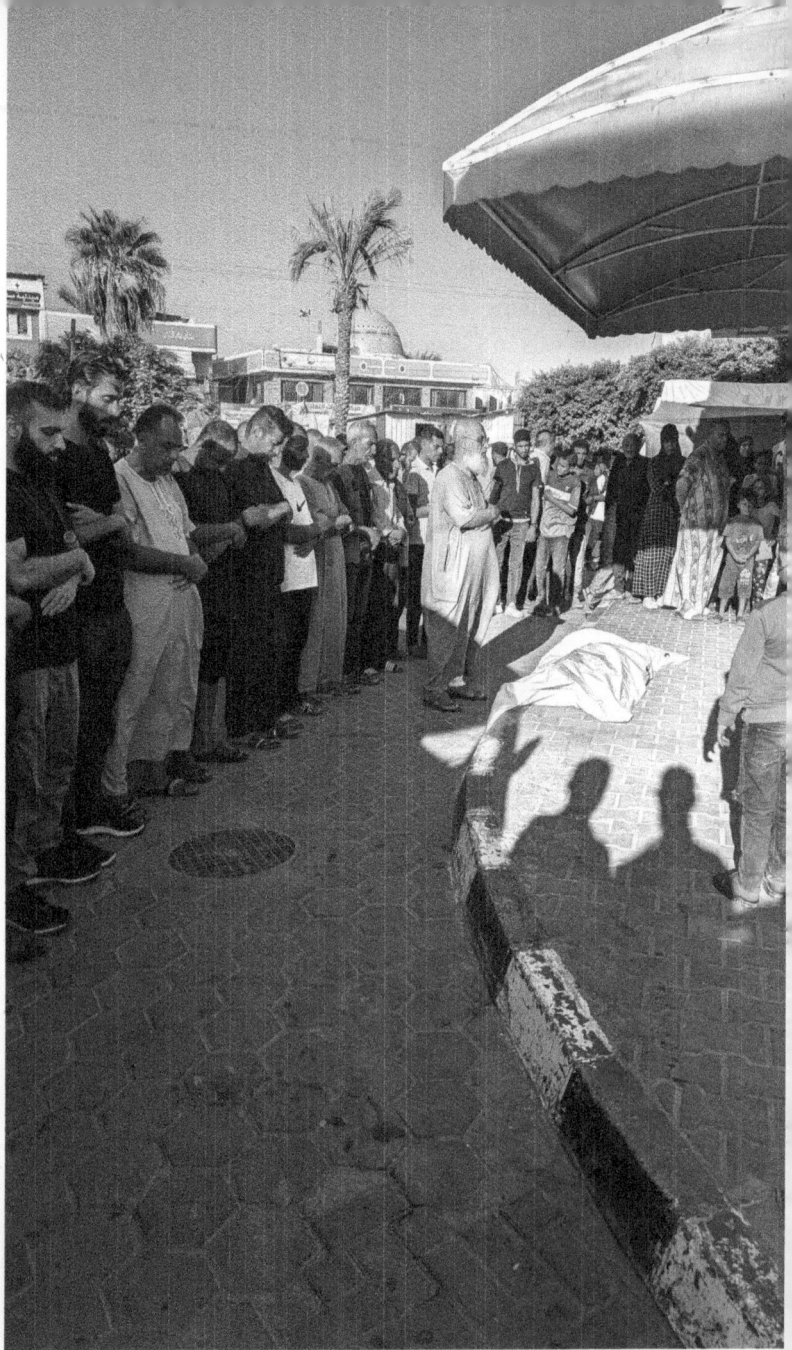

Janazah (funeral) prayers outside of the emergency department

Day 9
September 8 – Janazah

I don't think I need to set an alarm anymore. I'll just wait for the 5 am explosions to wake me up. Earlier this week, I wandered down to the ER after a late night explosion, and was told by the ER team to go back to sleep for it is extremely rare for overnight bombing victims to arrive in the emergency department immediately. There are reasons for this.

First, there has been a near complete destruction of the communication infrastructure between EMS (paramedics) and hospitals. Because of this, they often have to wait for the first victims to arrive in the hospital to find out what neighborhood to drive to.

Second, the Palestinian Red Crescent, who are responsible for field-to-hospital transfers, have been targeted especially at night, so the crews want to ensure there aren't continued operations at the blast site before they drive there. The combination of these factors plus the immense task of digging the rubble can often result in delays of up to six hours for an MCI to arrive at the hospital. To be clear, EMS are not afraid to go to the bombing sites, but once an aerial attack has started, their movements have to be precisely coordinated in order to mitigate the incredibly high risk they are taking. These workers are among the bravest people I have ever met.

We started the day with a mandatory update/briefing at the WHO office in Khan Yunis. It was attended by most of the emergency medical technicians (EMTs) from the various NGOs currently in Gaza. I've never been able to pay attention in these classroom settings, and coupled with fatigue, I ended up falling asleep for two hours. Luckily, Victoria paid attention and took notes for us.

A few of the important takeaways: There are currently only 64 EMTs in Gaza compared to the 160 just a few months ago. This is largely due to the limits that COGAT (the administrative arm of the Israeli military) has placed on the number of foreign aid workers they will process at the Allenby Crossing. This leaves NGOs competing for limited spots of longer durations, which is much more limiting than allowing a larger number of teams in and out of Gaza for 7–14 days as was the case when Rafah was open from December 29 to May 6.

Complicating this, an attack occurred at the Allenby Crossing yesterday so this access point will be closed until further notice. I hope it's just for a few days and not long-term because closing this crossing indefinitely will be the final death blow to Gaza.

Because we got back to the hospital late from the meeting, the schedule for the day got disrupted. When we finally arrived in the ER in the mid-afternoon, there were no traumas and most patients were relatively stable. Internet services were lost in all of Gaza for most of the day, which probably worked out well for me personally as I have become completely dependent on my medical apps to practice medicine. Israar and I went outside and ended up having a conversation with Hani Mahmoud, the head of Al Jazeera English in Gaza. It was an informal conversation where we learned about what he does and he shared some of his journalistic challenges. We're hoping to chat again over the coming days and weeks.

While chatting with him outside the ER entrance of Al Aqsa Hospital, a body draped in white cloth was brought to the steps of the ER, which has been the usual location of the *Janazah* (funeral prayers) for the deceased. This is the first *Janazah* I have attended in Gaza, and it was for a victim of one of yesterday's bombings. There were about 40 people who prayed over him in congregation. Before last year, there would have been thousands of people lining up to pray over this man and carry him through the streets for a final time before his burial. Due to the sheer number of deaths that have occurred, this wasn't the occasion it used to be, or should have been. After the prayer, the immediate family was allowed to unwrap his face to say their final farewell, and he was whisked into a nearby car to hopefully be buried at a local cemetery. I say "hopefully" because the people in attendance don't know where he actually will be buried. Because of the current death toll, Gaza is running out of places to bury people. The graves of people recently buried have been dug up and the new bodies have been piled on top of them, sometimes two to three in one grave. And in other instances I have been told about by journalists (I haven't seen it with my own eyes), people have been buried in the median separating roads, as well as the soft dirt next to sidewalks.

It turned out that the person buried today was a 41-year-old man—the exact same age as I am. You cannot, it seems, escape even the remembrance of your own mortality in this place.

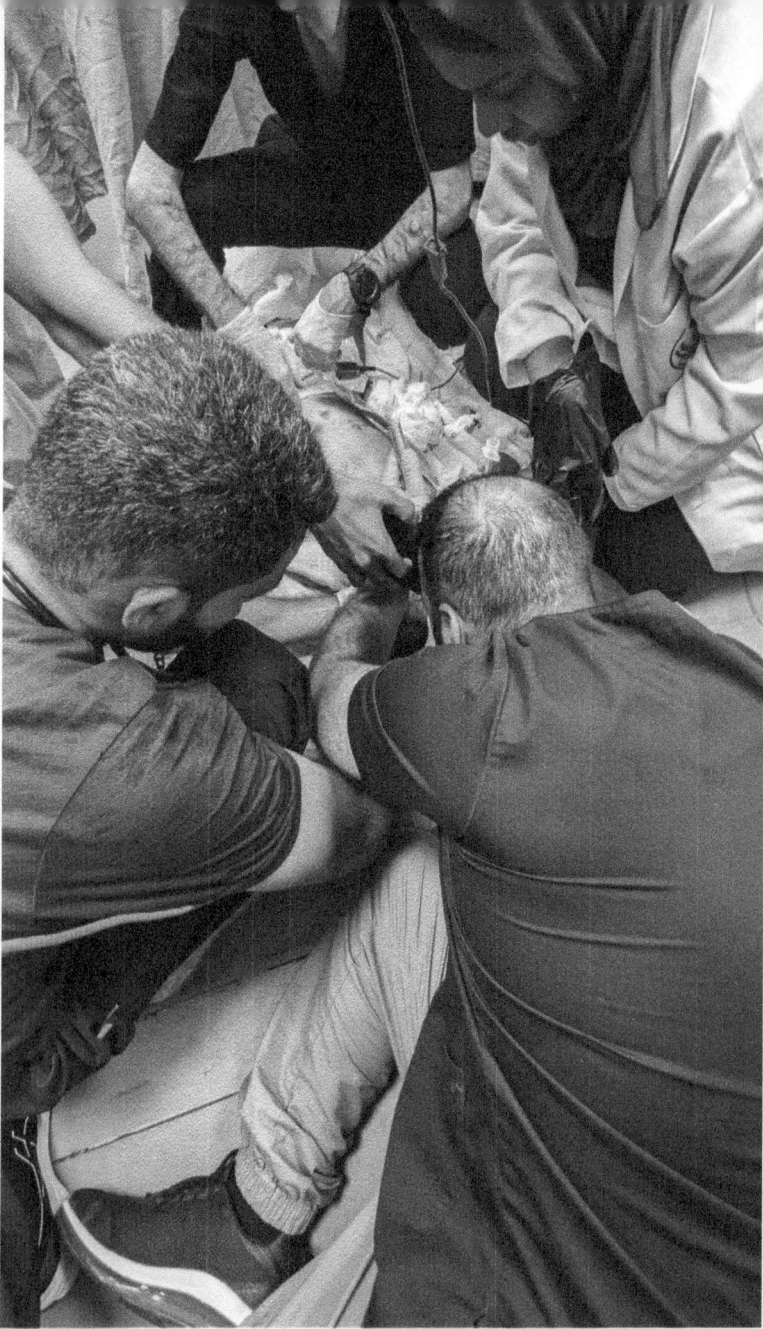

Dr. Israar Ul–Haq reviving a bombing victim on the floor of the emergency department

Day 10
September 9 – They Are NOT Okay

I turned 42 today. I'm not exactly sure why I'm starting today's entry by mentioning it, but somehow, it feels relevant. I've never really cared about my birthday, mostly preferring to be left alone or at least off the grid and using the time to just reflect in private. And since having kids, based on my wife's idea, we mostly use it as an excuse to visit my folks and say thanks to my mom and dad for raising me. It's the end of the day here and I just finished video calling my parents. Although I miss them, I'm exactly where I want to be today.

My first patient of the day was a 37-year-old from either the Nuseirat or Bureij displacement camps. She suffered a blast injury with burns worse than the children who died two days ago. This was greater than 90 percent total body surface area burns. Her eyes were filled with hardened soot and on close inspection, her corneas appeared melted (I don't have a better medical word to describe it). She was also bleeding internally from a severe pelvic injury. When the ICU physician arrived, he declared that this was a "hopeless case." I've heard this term repeatedly in my first week here.

Hopeless case. I've heard it used to describe cases of catastrophic head injury. But even though she was alive, burns so severe and covering such a large body surface area are a death sentence in Gaza. There's simply not enough gauze and antibiotics to prevent sepsis (systemic infection) and she will likely die within a few days.

I've been wrestling with how to present the Palestinians of Gaza in this journal. On the one hand, I have moments where I'm incredibly inspired and humbled by their resilience, strength and generosity. On the other hand, I worry about painting this unfair picture of them as heroes because I know they don't want to be heroes—they just want to live their lives and raise their children and families in peace. Labeling them as heroes also fails to convey the magnitude and sense of urgency needed to help change their condition. I've concluded that the ER waiting room is the ideal place to paint a picture of their current situation. The ER waiting room was the first on my list of things to write about when I arrived here, but so much has happened that I am now finally able to articulate what I have observed.

The ER at Al Aqsa Hospital treats between 1000 and 1200 patients per day, in an area that is less than half of my ER's size back home, which treats between 150 and 250 patients per day. Last year at this time, the ER in Gaza was seeing 600–700 patients per day.

The ER waiting room can only be described as CHAOS. Absolute chaos. It is a zoo, a madhouse. It is hot and humid because there is no air conditioning in the hospital and it's 35 degrees outside. There are patients and family members covering every part of the floor; most laying down or leaning against walls, and if they're lucky, some on stretchers. The crowd control is ineffective as it is staffed by mostly teenagers who have volunteered as hospital security. Often patients are accompanied by as many as 10–15 relatives who are standing over your shoulders and bumping into you during resuscitations.

You can't walk through the waiting room without being gently grabbed by patients and their family members asking for help. With my limited Arabic, I am occasionally able to help or direct them, or offer some medical assistance. But in most cases, I am reduced to saying to them *aj nabi* which means "foreigner" or *ana la atakalam al arabiyata* which means "I don't speak Arabic." When they hear this, they often smile, shake my hand and walk away. The doctors and nurses here in Gaza all speak English for the most part, so when you need a translator, you can easily get one.

One of the common reasons patients ask you for help is to review their results. There is no paper in the hospital and patients are handed their blood work results on small scraps of makeshift paper ripped from other things, and then they hand these to the doctor to review. They also take pictures of X-rays and ECGs on their phones and show them to you, often without any context and you have to try to figure out what to do next if you have a moment. And while you're standing in this sea of humanity trying to focus on one person, you are interrupted literally every minute by another seeking help. There is no break from this unless you go to the trauma room or leave the department altogether. It is non-stop.

This isn't how the system of flow was designed up until last year. This ER had an organized system and flow like any advanced ER around the world, but they have had to adapt their process so that when the next mass casualty of 10, 20 or 100 patients arrive, they are prepared to triage everyone and make the quick decisions of who can and cannot be saved.

In my first three days, I witnessed tensions between family members and staff escalate into full-on brawls, where family members had to be wrestled to the ground by nurses who escorted them out only to then return to work as if nothing happened. The first piece of advice that Israar gave me last week was to have my guard up at all times in the waiting room. Israar, who has seen the condition of the people change compared to his two previous visits, shared that there are many more cases of injuries to people they call "*mushkilat*," who are patients who have mostly suffered traumas related to fights for survival. In English they're also given the acronym BBO, which means "Beaten By Others." He also said he didn't see any suicide attempts on his previous visits but now these cases are on the rise.

Isn't this all contrary to the picture I've been painting of the Palestinians of Gaza being strong and resilient? Yes, they are indeed, especially at the moments of death and loss, but I believe one can be desperate and patient at the same time. They have been pushed way beyond the brink of what any human being should ever have to tolerate, and often arrive in the ER "triggered." When they're in the ER, it feels as if the entire world has turned their backs and abandoned them and they are in literal "fight or flight" mode. It becomes understandable why they feel the need to raise their voice to advocate for themselves or their sick loved ones.

Why couldn't I have just taken a two-minute video instead of writing all this? The people of Gaza, especially the women, have an incredible amount of something called "*Izza*," which can be translated as "honor." Imagine you're making a six-figure salary and then you've been homeless for a year, haven't bathed for months and aren't wearing your cleanest clothes and someone starts recording you. Just as you or I would probably say "please get that camera out of my face," they feel the same and are no different. Also, you really have to experience the chaos, claustrophobia and desperation of the ER waiting room to truly understand it; it is not something that could ever translate well to video. Lastly, people don't see the utility in recording their suffering anymore. It's been a year and everyone in the world has seen the footage. In their mind (and mine), if the first video or picture of a headless or charred baby didn't motivate the world to act, I doubt the thousandth will either.

I write all this to say that these people are NOT okay. They could not be further from being okay. They are in desperate need of food, water, shelter, safety, dignity and medical attention. And this doesn't include the daily threat of bombings without relief in sight. The best way to describe them is that they are desperate for relief, and continue to "carry on," because that is all they CAN do. Even in the past week, I've witnessed the hospital stairwells and hallways filling with makeshift tents as an increasing number of people are returning from the mid-August evacuation. The area was deemed safe by the IDF ten days ago but most people lack trust and aren't returning until they are sure it is the best place for them due to the incredible difficulty in moving whatever is left of their life and families again and again.

Speaking to the director of the ER today, Dr. Haddad, he expects three to five hundred thousand people to return to the region in the next few weeks which will likely increase the ER volumes to 1500–1600 patients per day, creating another humanitarian crisis within the already stretched hospital that he is desperately scrambling to solve before it begins.

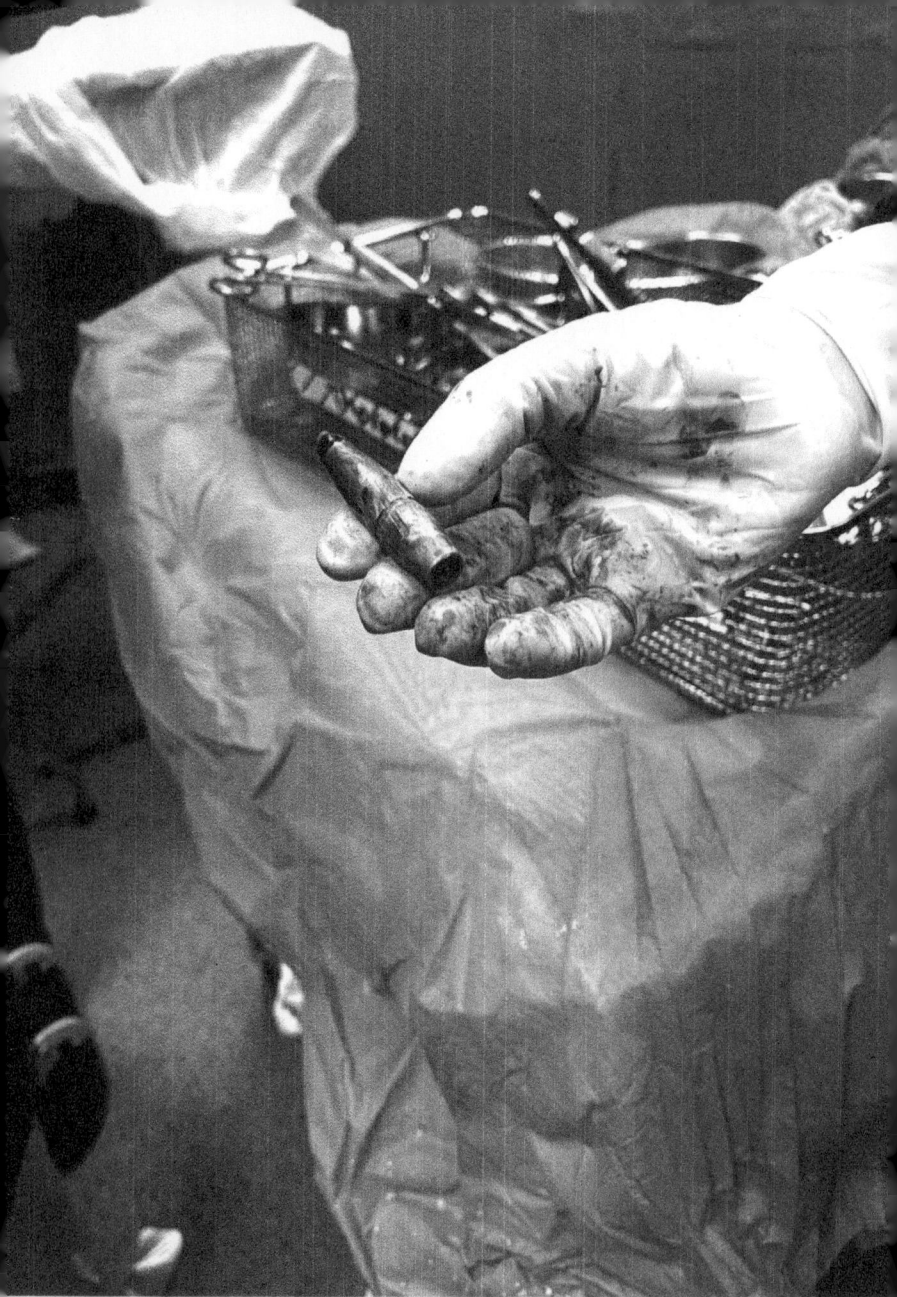

A quadcopter bullet removed from a patient in the operating room; photo credit, Dr. Victoria Aveson

Day 11
September 10 – Quadcopter

Today was the busiest day for mass casual incidents since we arrived, but it was not what I would consider a bad day anymore. Much of the talk in the department was about the 2000-pound bomb that was dropped on the Al Mawasi camp, but we never received any of their casualties because we were told most of the victims were either buried in the sand or evaporated. Despite all of the injured having a long and painful path to recovery, everyone we treated was alive at the end of the day, so that is a win.

The day started with a 48-year-old man named Ayman who was shot by an IDF quadcopter and suffered wounds to his chest and left leg. A father of two boys and three girls, he is a tomato farmer in his neighborhood of Musaddar Village. He was shocked over what happened because he says the IDF knows him well. But as he was walking back home after farming on his small plot of land, the quadcopter began firing at him without warning and dropped grenades that missed him. This man's home is in the IDF-designated safe zone.

When talking to several staff here, many describe the quadcopters as the weapon they fear more than bombs. Regarding the bombs, they say that the one you hear is not the one you have to worry about. The bomb you didn't hear is the one that killed you. The quadcopters are equipped with speakers that shout warnings and instructions, and armed with grenades and exploding bullets. As one physician explained, if you are struck with one of these bullets, it is an "automatic amputation." I don't believe this to be a dramatization as both times I've been outdoors and a quadcopter approached, people were quick to scatter and look for cover.

The morning and early afternoon were relatively quiet, so Israar and I visited our favorite spot on the balcony of the ICU to catch a breeze and stare out over Gaza. Suddenly, a loud explosion from about 500 m away startled us, and we knew that patients would be arriving shortly. We made our way down to the ER where four-year-old Yusuf awaited us. He had a traumatic head injury with an extensive, "degloved" scalp injury. He was alert, crying, covered in the usual ash and coughing up frothy/bloody secretions that were foaming at his mouth. He was all alone and through his secretions continued to repeatedly cry "Baba! Baba!" hoping his father would arrive to comfort him. We thought he looked stable, but within 30 seconds he suddenly stopped crying and went limp and his face went pale. We could barely feel a pulse, and immediately began chest compressions, inserted a breathing tube, and cut the left side of his chest to insert a chest drain. After about 45 minutes, his vitals improved and his test results revealed the worst lung contusion I've ever seen. When his father finally arrived, he was angry and in tears screaming, "does he look like a fighter?!" to anyone who would listen. He eventually calmed down and took his place at his son's side until he was moved to the ICU. We checked on him several hours later and he appeared to be stable, but I still can't get that cry of "Baba" out of my head, when his father wasn't there. That's how my four-year-old son refers to me, and I hear his voice in Yusuf's cries. I confirmed that Yusuf's home is also in the designated safe zone.

Just as Yusuf was being stabilized, we received seven more patients with blast injuries, two of whom were severe enough for the resuscitation room. Of the seven in total, three were children under the age of six with severe limb injuries. Just to describe the chaos, five of these patients were treated on the floor of the waiting room. It's wild to think that a three-year-old with a bone and vascular injury to her arm wasn't considered injured enough to make it into our resuscitation rooms.

One of the injuries was a gaping forearm injury, where the tendons, muscles and vessels were all exposed and needed a vascular surgeon, as we couldn't control the bleeding. Two doctors arrived, a retired general surgeon and a younger vascular surgeon. The older general surgeon jumped in and the vascular surgeon backed off, whispering to me "I should be the one fixing this but he's older and I have to respect him." Near the end of the repair, while the general surgeon was singing *nasheeds* (Islamic songs typically sung in Arabic), he did an incredibly skilled thing with the wound, and could tell I was impressed. He looked up at me with the side glance, winked and said, "they didn't teach you this in Canada?"

After all these patients were sorted out, I sat on the steps of the courtyard of the hospital to get some fresh air. My friend, nurse Saeed, sat with me and began telling me the story of how he has lost parents, his brother, his sister, and his five-year-old daughter, Dema in the last year. I asked him how he carries on, and he said, "everything that is decreed for me is good and I accept it with happiness." Before we could finish our conversation, another loud explosion was heard in the distance.

Israar called me back to the trauma room where we waited for the next MCI to arrive. In Canada, whenever we get notified of a trauma, we usually receive 10–15-minute advanced notice at which point the entire team organizes ourselves around an empty bed, gets fully dressed in our personal protective equipment including gowns, gloves and a mask, and a face shield, and then waits for the paramedics to arrive with the patient. We all have our assigned roles and know exactly where we'll be standing next to the bedside. Each nurse knows their specific responsibility during the resuscitation. In Gaza, most critical patients arrive in the trauma bay suddenly, with no warning and we have to act immediately, often working on our hands and knees.

The final mass casualty of the day were two sisters and their uncle. Five-year-old Aseel and nine- year-old Ghazal were covered in shrapnel from head to toe, with tiny pieces embedded all over their skin. All three of them had multiple limb fractures. Their 32-year-old uncle suffered the most severe injuries and needed to be sent to the OR. Compared to the patients that I've seen over the last couple of days, these patients were awake and relatively stable, despite the fact that they will still have a long recovery.

Near the end of our work, Aseel and Ghazal's grandmother arrived. Crying, she said, "Ghazal, your mom is dead." Without any emotion or hesitation, the nine-year-old calmly replied, "I know."

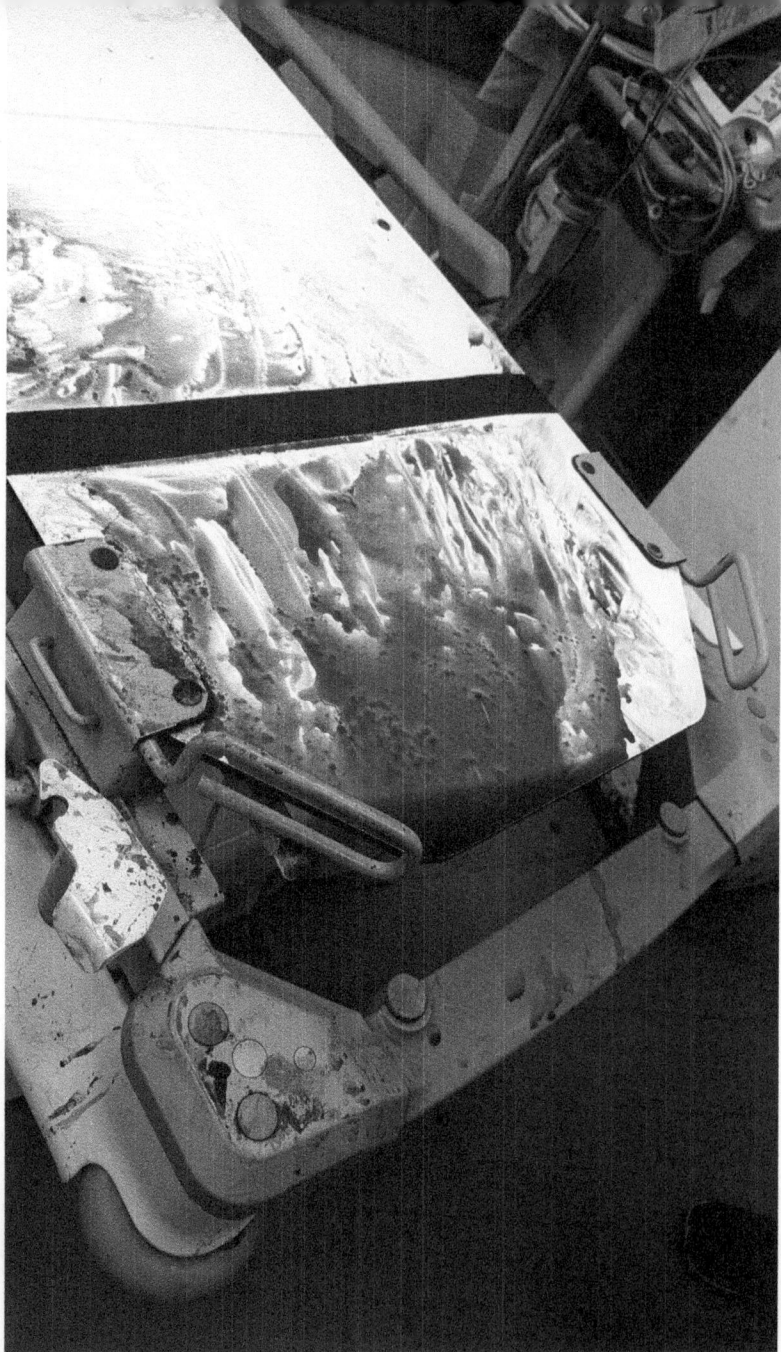

Red Zone stretcher, after a mass casualty incident (MCI)

Day 13
September 12 – Red Zone

I wasn't able to journal yesterday because as soon as I started writing (around 11 pm) an explosion shook the window and doors of our room. I estimated it was less than 500 m away, so I assumed casualties would be arriving soon, so I changed into scrubs again and ran down to the ER and waited on the front steps where there was a nice breeze. After 45 minutes, no one had arrived so I went back upstairs to sleep. Every single time a bomb explodes, I start imagining what might arrive in order to mentally prepare, and every time a casualty does arrive it's something I wasn't expecting.

I think I might be finally starting to hit my stride here. This isn't something I ever took for granted in the days and weeks leading up to my arrival. After 15 years of emergency medicine work, I have complete trust and belief in my skills, but I know I was entering a foreign land, a hospital with a completely different culture and language, in an extremely low resource setting. Early in my career, I used to be a trauma instructor, but in Gaza, I certainly would not be the expert in trauma. I even imagined myself saying to them, "I'm good at trauma" and the Palestinian doctors replying like Bane in *The Dark Knight Rises* (replacing darkness with trauma): "You merely adopted trauma. We were born in it … molded by it."

As I mentioned earlier, only two of the 40 ER physicians at Al Aqsa Hospital are board certified (many more would be if not for the circumstances). So, whenever I'm introduced by someone, it is as "this is Dr. Salman, *consultant* ER physician," which automatically gains me some credibility with whoever I was just introduced to. The "consultant" level is the equivalent of "attending" back home. The reason I bring this up is that it is really apparent how much everyone here values education and achieving a milestone in education, which I'll hopefully cover when I write about the destruction of the universities and academic institutions here in Gaza.

Despite this respect that being board certified earns me, it is very clear that many of the ER physicians I have worked alongside here are vastly superior clinicians to me in many ways. It has been humbling but also motivating to try to prove myself and earn their trust, and I think it finally started to happen this past week.

The ER is divided into three zones. The Red Zone is the advanced trauma, critical care and resuscitation zone (it's where the sickest patients go). The Yellow Zone is the acute monitoring zone for patients who do not require immediate life-saving interventions. And the Green Zone is their minor treatment and intermediate zone, in a tent just outside the entrance of the ER. There's also a dedicated suturing zone and a separate pediatric ER/urgent care. Earlier this week, after working together on a number of resuscitations together, Dr. Haddad requested that Israar and I only work in the Red Zone, which is incredibly flattering coming from a man of his stature, skills and a person I have come to admire greatly. The other ER physicians have also welcomed us as colleagues and equals. We were never here to lead, but rather to lend a helping set of skilled hands. Perhaps it is my own corrupt heart that had me believing they might think "We don't need these Western doctors to help us," because every single one of them has welcomed us and thanked us, and said that we are part of their family and they consider us their brothers. I'm very glad that my stay here is for one month. If I were here for only two weeks, I'd be leaving just as I was getting comfortable, but now I feel like I have another three weeks of being a useful member of the team.

What is it like resuscitating a patient in the Red Zone? The room is 15x20 ft, and humid, unlike the chilly air-conditioned resuscitation rooms back home. There are three stretchers but during the worst of the killing there have been times where up to ten patients were all on the floor beside each other. The room is a third the size of the room we use for two patients back in Canada.

The first thing I notice every day is that the room is thick with the smell of blood. There are permanent blood stains on the curtains, stretchers, and most reusable and permanent furniture. No matter what cleaning solution is used, the room always smells like blood. It's taken nine days of working between 10 and 14 hours per day, and I think I'm finally becoming nose-blind to the smell. This is probably one of the memories that will take the longest to fade.

The curtains separating stretchers are held up by zip ties attached to the ceiling, and there are several spots on the ceiling where water leaks onto your head while you work on patients. This is an incredible pain when you're performing a procedure and your glasses get wet.

Once a patient is suddenly carried in and placed on the floor, you spring into action. But just as you start, their small room gets filled with security, 5–10 family members, and photojournalists trying to get a picture of the injuries. There have been several instances of fights between media and family/security, who don't want pictures taken of their loved ones in this state, that have jostled the stretcher where the patient lay.

Most of these trauma cases involve multiple casualties, so the room gets filled with three patients on stretchers or the floor, five ER doctors, six to eight nurses, security, surgeons and multiple family members. This means there can be up to 30 people in this 15x30-ft space during a mass casualty incident.

There's no paper, so you rely on everyone's memory to tell you what medication was given and at what time, or you write critical information on the patient's skin. And you often have an audience of several family members literally over your shoulder or at your waist while you insert a breathing or chest tube in their child.

Speaking of procedures, there is NO sterility to any of these emergent procedures. No cleaning solution, no sterile drapes, gowns or gloves, and no masks. You just spray some saline on the area and cut the skin. I've inserted central venous catheters into femoral veins while on the floor, which are nearly guaranteed to become infected. And the one thing I can't seem to ignore is the tens of flies that land on your skin and the patient's skin the entire time. It's no wonder that so many patients have had to return to the OR after surgeries to have their wounds cleaned of the maggots that have accumulated inside them.

By the time the resuscitation is complete (which is ideally less than 45 minutes when they go to the operating room or move to another ward), the floor is covered in blood. More blood than I've seen in my career. Just when I thought I was going nose-blind to the smell of blood, the fresh blood gets in your nose again. By the end of the case, you are drenched in sweat and often have your scrubs stained with blood. You try to rinse parts of it off because there's no point in changing until the end of the day.

Then, while housekeeping mops the floor, the team that remains sits along the walls of the room, and takes a breather while they wait for the next one to arrive.

At 10 pm today, a nearby explosion brought three patients to the Red Zone: a seven-year-old boy with a shrapnel injury to his abdomen (he lived), a 64-year-old lady with a catastrophic head injury who died in the ER, and a 25-year-old man with complete amputations of his left and right legs above the knees. His left leg was completely blown off and his right leg was only attached by skin soft tissue and vessels, and his family was refusing to allow an amputation, until the leg was uncovered and even a non-medical person could understand there was no saving it. The thing that caught my eye is that on the floor of the room next to him was an olive branch stained with blood. I don't know how it got there, but I couldn't find a more perfect metaphor for what is happening here. If this man lives, I can't even imagine how difficult his life will be. There are very few wheelchair ramps in Gaza or even wheelchairs. Any disability infrastructure has been severely damaged and it will be nearly impossible to get anywhere without having a loved one carry you around (and that's if you still have caregivers who are alive).

Once the patient left the Red Zone and was moved to the OR, Dr. Wasim, one of the ER physicians involved, turned to me and said, "He is my friend. He lives next door to me, and he is alone."

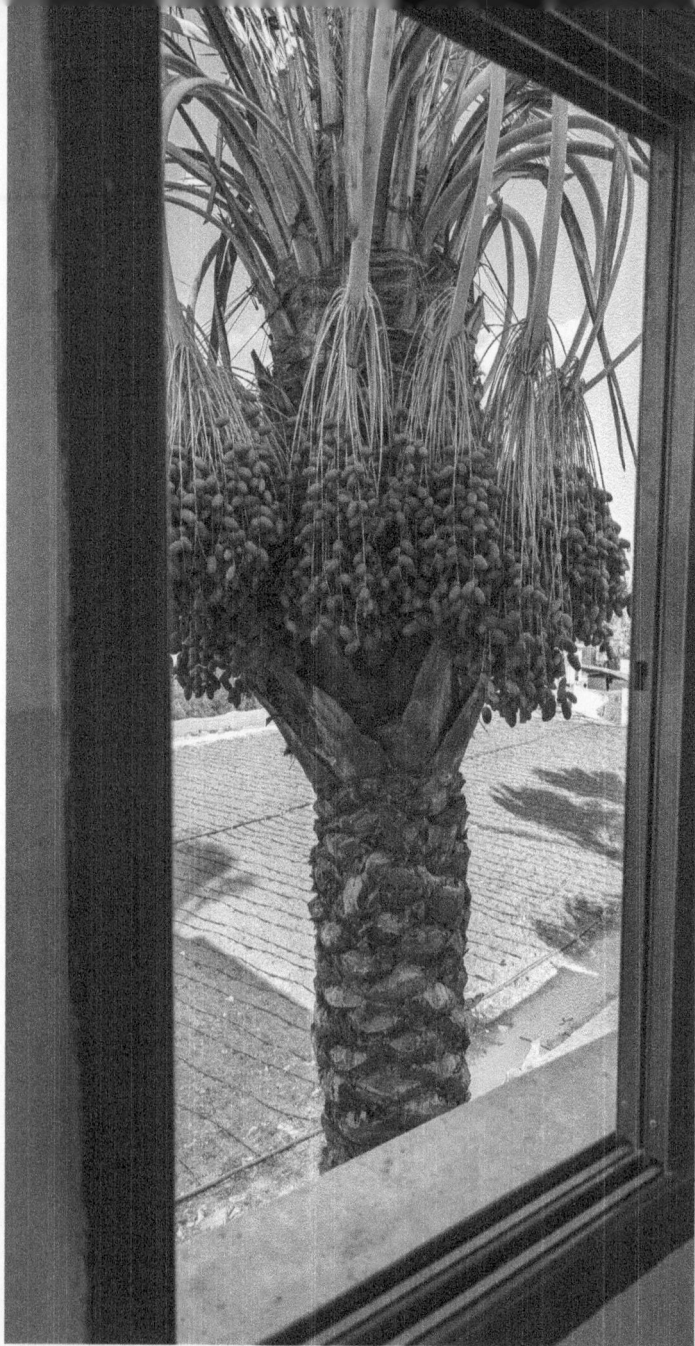

Date Palm outside of Al Aqsa Martyrs Mosque,
Deir Al Balah, Gaza

Day 15
September 14 – Palestine Was a Paradise

A few updates: The 37-year-old female with burns to >90 percent of her body from September 9 is dead.

The four-year-old boy Yusuf, with the lung contusions, is alive and continuing to recover. I ran into his father in between the emergency department and the ICU and he grabbed my shoulder and gave me an update and shared how *mashkoor* (thankful) he was with our care. When we visited Yusuf in the ICU, he still had a breathing tube, but his eyes were open and he looked much better. As part of my work, I'm trying to focus and find meaning in the process and not solely on the outcomes, given how much death has occurred despite our best efforts. I have to admit that its encouraging and motivating to see a child on his way to making a complete recovery.

I wasn't able to journal last night for the same reason I didn't write two nights ago. At 10:30 pm, an explosion occurred in very close proximity to the hospital, to the degree that it shook even the emergency department. Even the staff who are accustomed to these events went "whoa." An hour later, two casualties arrived: a man and woman, both in their late 20s.

The man suffered burns to >60 percent of his body. In most of these cases, we've been told to not insert a breathing tube into these patients as the mortality is exceptionally high and that the ICU would reject any patient with burns >30 percent of their total body surface area. However, in this case, the ICU had open beds and the intensivist came down and helped secure a breathing tube and admit to the ICU.

The woman, presumably related (there was no family present to confirm), had severe bleeding into her abdomen and chest, so we began transfusing her with blood, inserted a chest tube, and rushed her to the operating room. It was 1 am when this event concluded and it was time to sleep.

Today, our team agreed to take a day off and visit a guest house 20 minutes away to have our first shower and rest. At the last minute, we were notified that we did not get clearance from the IDF and our route was not safe. It being too risky to leave the hospital, we just decided to work today.

The loudest explosion we heard today occurred at the Maghazi camp, where a bomb landed on a tent. Two victims arrived in the emergency department and they were pronounced dead in the waiting room. They were removed very quickly so I didn't get the chance to examine and explore the full extent of their injuries and cause of death, but they appeared to be burnt and had severe crushed head injuries.

It's been two weeks, and something I feared is beginning to happen. I'm starting to view and remember these patients more by their injuries, and less as complete human beings with families and complex, beautiful lives. I'm trying very hard to learn their names, their family, who they were, and what they did, but in the chaos of the waiting and resuscitation rooms, it is often the last thing I'm able to ask. I suppose this is all part of the dehumanization of the Palestinians, that if after witnessing only two weeks of death and gruesome injuries has caused me to lose sight of my goal, I can understand how an entire year of media coverage can numb people into simply swiping to the next video or picture in their algorithm. Have I become desensitized to this violence? Has my heart hardened? Or have I just succeeded in compartmentalizing what I've experienced in a healthy manner? I honestly don't know at the moment, and will take time to come to an answer.

Today our friend and handler for our mission, Dr. Fowzi (the man we met on our arrival in Gaza) found us falafel sandwiches from a street vendor and a handful of grapes. He told us about how over 50 varieties of grapes used to grow in Gaza, before over 96 percent of farmland was destroyed (according to the UN Trade and Development Agency). He had a large farm with over 600 trees that grew several varieties of oranges including the Pakistani "kinnoo," pears, guavas, lemons, grapefruit, figs, olives, dates and some exotic fruit that he showed us pictures of, but we still have no idea what they are. At age 49, he's worked incredibly hard his entire life and despite the hardships of the occupation, he said he lived a good life. "We used to be rich ... and now we are not."

Dr. Fowzi completed his PhD in The Sudan, and his Bachelor's and Master's degrees at the NED University in Karachi, Pakistan. He speaks better Urdu than I do, and he likes to tease me calling me "*yaar*," which means "buddy" in Urdu. Myself and Victoria don't eat a lot, so he says hilarious things like when our families see how skinny we've become, they will think he is a "*kanjoos aadmi*," which means "cheapskate." I've known this man for less than two weeks, but I love him dearly and thinking about parting from him in just over two weeks fills me with an incredible sadness.

I asked him what remains of his farm and he replied, "They destroyed all of my trees." Our conversation concluded with him staring in the distance like he was picturing something and saying "Palestine was like paradise."

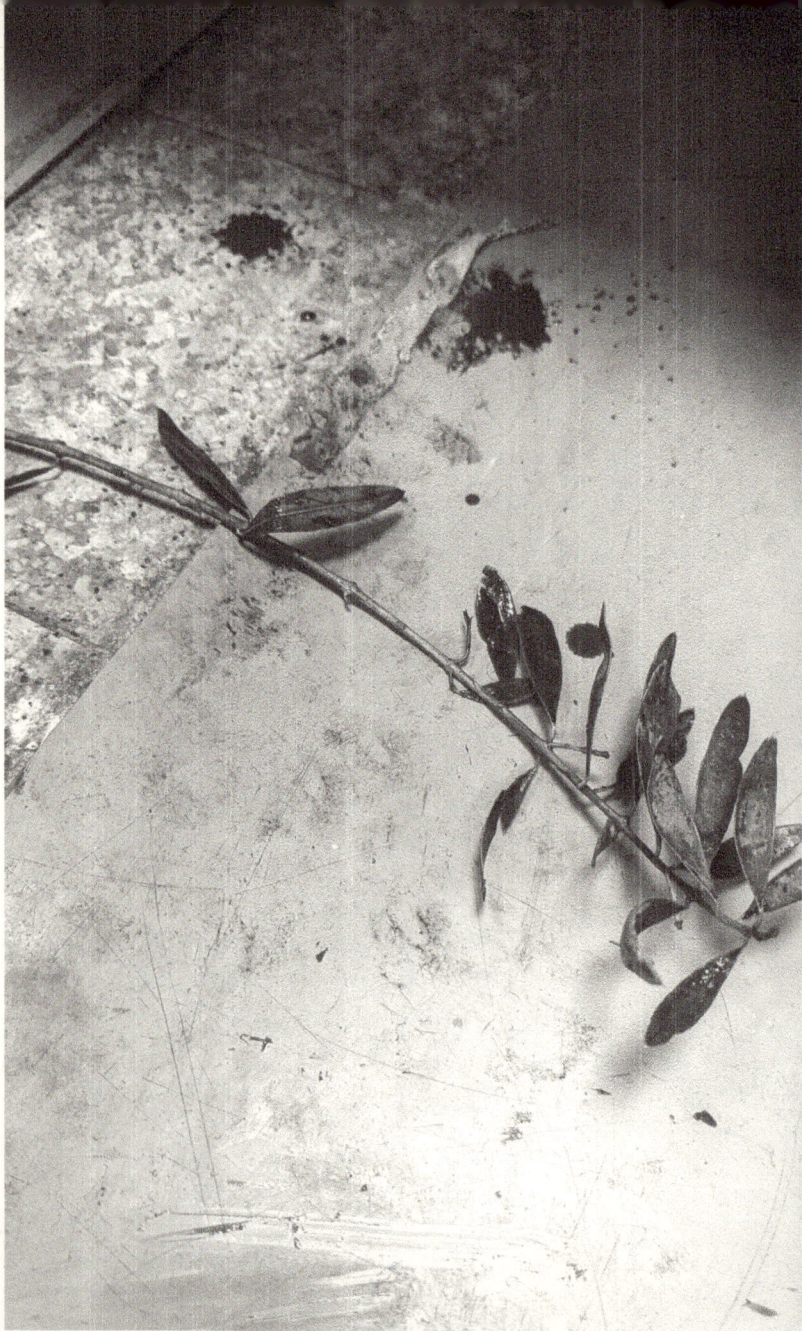

An olive branch stained with blood on the floor of the emergency department

Day 17
September 16 – No One Is Unaffected

Forgiveness in advance, for this entry will contain two detailed descriptions of injuries to the male and female reproductive organs. It's not intended for shock value, but there are a few observations I need to remind myself of.

Our first trauma patient of the day was Abdul Rahman, a 31-year-old male from Nuseirat. According to those who know him, he's responsible for helping to supply water from a water distribution vehicle to the people in his displacement camp. The witnesses from today said that he was helping people fill their water containers when a bomb landed near him. When he arrived, his left leg was completely blown off and he had extensive bone and soft tissue loss at the level of his right ankle. Because the hospital has run out of sterile gauze and other surgical supplies, he had to be transferred to a nearby field hospital for a double leg amputation. Due to the blast, he also suffered a very significant injury to his genitals. There was shrapnel embedded everywhere in his penis, and it was markedly swollen, bruised, and bleeding at multiple sites. It was nearly impossible to recognize anatomic landmarks and he was also bleeding due to a suspected urethral injury. Our urologist inserted a catheter and plans on exploring his injuries in the operating room.

The second notable injury was a teenage boy in the waiting room, who had a shrapnel injury to his chest and bleeding surrounding his heart who wasn't considered critical enough to make it to the Red Zone. He was treated and sent to the OR from the waiting room, without even getting a stretcher. The thoracic surgeon saw me later on and showed me a video of the gush of blood that was released after making the incision to the membrane of his heart. He is alive and recovering.

The final "notable" (I hate using this word, but can't find a better one) patient was a man in his 20s who suffered a blast injury that amputated his right foot and caused a cat-astrophic head injury with exposed brain matter. He was stabilized and taken to the ICU where he will likely die. During this man's resuscitation, I observed an interesting thing. A volunteer physician on the neurosurgery team was receiving condolences from nearly everyone he met. When I asked what was going on, Dr. Khalil told me that this man's brother died in a bombing today, and that he's still continu-ing his duty at work.

For about the 20th time this trip, I've asked a question that I knew the answer to, but needed to hear directly from a Palestinian. "Why is he still working today?" A few of the nurses explained: "Everyone here has lost multiple people. There isn't a single person in Gaza who is untouched by this. Every time we come to work, we worry our family will be bombed. Every time we hear a bomb, we wonder if it hit our neighborhood or our home."

I was well aware before I arrived that everyone in Gaza has been touched by this conflict. Working side by side with these doctors and nurses every day, it's so easy to forget that they all live in tents and have suffered immeasurable loss, yet they still show up to work with good nature, treat each other like best friends and work extremely hard and professionally, despite carrying these losses and empty spaces with them. If you didn't know what was happening in Gaza and just spent the day with the staff (ignoring the regular mass casualties), you would never be able to guess what's happening here by examining their demeanor.

The nurses then pointed to a nurse named Ghaleb, who entered the Red Zone singing, and who several described as "the teddy bear of the department." "He has lost 57 family members."

I don't bring this up as some sort of "wow, look at the triumph of the human spirit," but this is more of a reminder to myself because it's so easy to forget. I'm writing this during a quiet moment in the ER and I'm watching three nurses tease each other and joke around like they have dinner plans later. They're not plotting revenge and I haven't heard any of them even say a hateful thing. It's just friends messing around with each other.

Catching up with Victoria, she shared with me some of the things she's been witnessing: In North America, when people get a colostomy or ileostomy after a cancer resection (or more often in Gaza, a trauma surgery), she's accustomed to patients changing their colostomy bag three or more times a day. In Gaza, you get one colostomy bag, and that's your bag. Forever. When the clips and the sticky part of the bag no longer stick to your body and become loose, she has seen patients tie a string around their abdomen to try and keep it in place. Another observation from Victoria is that Gaza also has no radiation therapy due to the absurd fear that bringing radioactive materials into Gaza will be used to create a nuclear weapon.

What I have also noticed personally is that there are no urinary catheter bags in Gaza. So when we insert them, we're sending patients home with catheters attached to chest tube bottles. I have also seen patients walking in the waiting room of the ER with the end of their catheter tube taped to an empty 2-L bottle of water.

The case Victoria is particularly invested in is a woman in her late 20s, who suffered an explosive injury to her perineum a week ago. The perineum is the anatomic area between your rectum and your external genitalia. Victoria described this injury to me as though the bomb hit the ground and exploded, and then the force of the blast went up from the ground and into this woman's pelvis, leaving a gaping opening where her genitalia would be as well as her rectum, bladder and pelvis. Trying not to be crude in any way, but also at a loss for how exactly to describe it in a manner that I could visualize and describe to show the viciousness of the injury, Victoria said that the bladder catheter has been placed into an opening in her pelvis that looks like raw meat. This is clearly a life-altering injury for this young patient. There are two key points I wanted to share from this patient.

First, there are so many different types of weapons being used on the Palestinians in Gaza and the medical staff have become adept at being able to tell what type of weapon is used in a mass casualty. The same bombs that amputate legs also appear to cause significant pelvic and rectal injuries because the force is from the ground upwards, usually when they're dropped on tents. When other bombs land on the few remaining viable concrete structures left, they cause crush injuries to the head, chest and limbs. There are also rockets and missiles that explode in the air causing a blast of force and heat that create a pressure difference between the abdomen/chest and the atmosphere, rupturing organs without causing significant external bleeding (these ones can be difficult to detect). And then, of course, there appear to be weapons that are just meant to cause burns. I'm by no means a weapons expert, but it does feel like there are days with themes similar to my usual ER shift. For example, some shifts in the ER feel like chest pain days and other shifts feel like abdominal pain days. But everyone I talked to in the hospital feels like the weapons being used on them change week to week. Some weeks, the casualties suffer burns, and some weeks or days, all the casualties appear to be maimed with exploding bullets to the limbs from the quadcopters. The prevailing sentiment amongst the medical staff is that they believe they are subjects in an inhumane and cruel experiment and that they're seeing injury patterns they have not witnessed in any previous IDF attacks. I'm trying my best to be diligent and chart these injury patterns to see if a trend can be established by the end of the month. I'm hoping this is also being recorded by others as well.

The second point of interest about this young woman is that Victoria is trying her best to medevac (medical evacuation) her to another country. The staff have done an admirable job of managing her dressing changes, but this young woman desperately needs major reconstructive surgery at an academic institution to repair her bladder, urinary tract and reproductive organs. The first step in this process is to add her name to a Ministry of Health list, which can be incredibly difficult, because finding something as basic as the patient ID number is onerous. There are no paper records and the computer health informatics system has been destroyed. This list is then shared with the Israeli Administration. After a lengthy and often arbitrary process of receiving security clearance from the IDF, the various countries involved in medevacs (e.g. UAE, Egypt) can sign up and agree to take her (if/when that clearance ever occurs). There isn't much clarity on how long this process will take, whether it's days, weeks or months. When I know more, I hope to update this journal.

This brings me to a topic I had no intention of writing about but now feel compelled to after all that I've seen and heard thus far. It would be ideal to transfer complex patients to the Al-Shifa Medical Center, an institution of specialization within Gaza that may have been able to offer advanced treatments and operations like the one this patient needs.

Al Aqsa Hospital, Deir Al Balah, Gaza

Day 18
September 17 – House of Healing

There existed a place in Gaza that was an immense source of pride for everyone that lived here. It was a place that I've heard many hospital staff refer to as the "heart of Gaza." This place was Al-Shifa Hospital in Gaza City. Translated from Arabic "*Al-Shifa*" means "The Cure." I say "was" because in April of 2024 the IDF conducted a siege of the hospital (that siege was condemned by several well-known and respected global humanitarian organizations) leaving the hospital in ruins and permanently closed. Many hospital workers told me: "I didn't cry when my home was destroyed but I cried while they destroyed Al-Shifa."

The reason I feel compelled to write about it is that I've encountered so many people at Al Aqsa Hospital who used to work at Al-Shifa who had to find new hospitals for employment.

Al-Shifa Hospital was founded in 1946 in Palestine and expanded during the Egyptian and Israeli occupations. Ironically, it was during the Israeli occupation in the 1980s that it received one of its most significant expansions and architectural upgrades. It was transferred to the Palestinian Authority following the signing of the Oslo Accords in 1994, and was again expanded with new buildings, creating a sprawling multi-building campus. The capacity of the hospital was 720 beds, and it employed over 1500 people, including 500 doctors and over 750 nurses and support staff.

To provide context to my medical colleagues as to the scope of services offered here, they used to perform cardiac surgery, cardiac catheterization and endovascular therapy for hyperacute ischemic strokes and housed one of the only two MRI machines in all of Gaza. The resuscitation zone of the ER alone had 14 beds! (My hospital back home has three.) The ER was massive and even when you look at old pictures of the atrium and the foyer, it looked like a high-end hotel and not a hospital (I encourage you to look up the before pictures). Without exaggeration, Al-Shifa would not have been out of place when standing next to some of the greatest hospitals in North America and Europe.

The reason I share all this is because I really can't completely illustrate the full scope of limitations to providing care in Gaza without mentioning the destruction of the Al-Shifa Hospital.

On September 14th, we received a 49-year-old female named Rajab who suffered a cardiac arrest after a massive heart attack. She got her pulse back without a long delay, and her ECG showed changes that would normally indicate she needed an urgent cardiac stent. One year ago, she would have been transferred to Al-Shifa for this procedure without hesitation, but instead remained at our hospital to be treated with whatever scarce resources we had available. There is now an increased likelihood of a very young patient's heart suffering more damage which could have been prevented.

Another example is of a young male in his 40s who suffered a stroke who could have been transferred to Al-Shifa for endovascular therapy and a chance of regaining his right hand and leg function. But he will now live the rest of his life with weakness to the entire right side of his body.

It's been six months since Al-Shifa was left in ruins and even when nurses and doctors who used to work there talk about it, their eyes well up and they get quite emotional. My friend and colleague here, an ER doctor named Anwar who once worked at Al-Shifa, put it this way: "Once the IDF destroyed Al-Shifa, that was the moment I knew we had no control over our fate." I also had the chance to meet Dr. Munir, a senior ER physician at Al-Shifa (and the other board-certified ER physician at my hospital) who was arbitrarily imprisoned for five months at Ofer Prison in the Israeli-occupied West Bank last November, during the first siege of Al-Shifa. He said he was "hit in the head many times" and that the IDF "threatened to kill me." He was never charged with any crimes and was released as unceremoniously as he was detained. He now works as an ER consultant at Al Aqsa Hospital.

Whenever I hear these stories, I keep returning to the thought of how our medical community, medical establishments and society as a whole would have reacted to the razing of our finest institutions of healing. I imagine what would happen if the Ottawa Heart Institute or the Mayo Clinic were destroyed and many of the professors and great medical academics we learned from were imprisoned without any just cause. How would we have collectively reacted?

I believe in the sanctity of medical institutions and places of healing, and breaches of this sanctity have occurred in a manner that has never occurred in history on such a scale as it has occurred in Gaza. Al-Shifa is only one of several hospitals which have permanently closed due to the destruction of the buildings. Al-Shifa (and these other hospitals) should have been the tipping point for our medical establishments to finally stand in solidarity with the doctors, nurses and vulnerable patients in Gaza. This unfortunately has not yet happened and I believe it is a failure of humanity that we will regret when the world finally views this conflict with a different lens five, ten, or twenty years from now.

It is clear to me from everyone I've spoken to that Al-Shifa Hospital was the medical heart of Gaza, and that heart is now shattered.

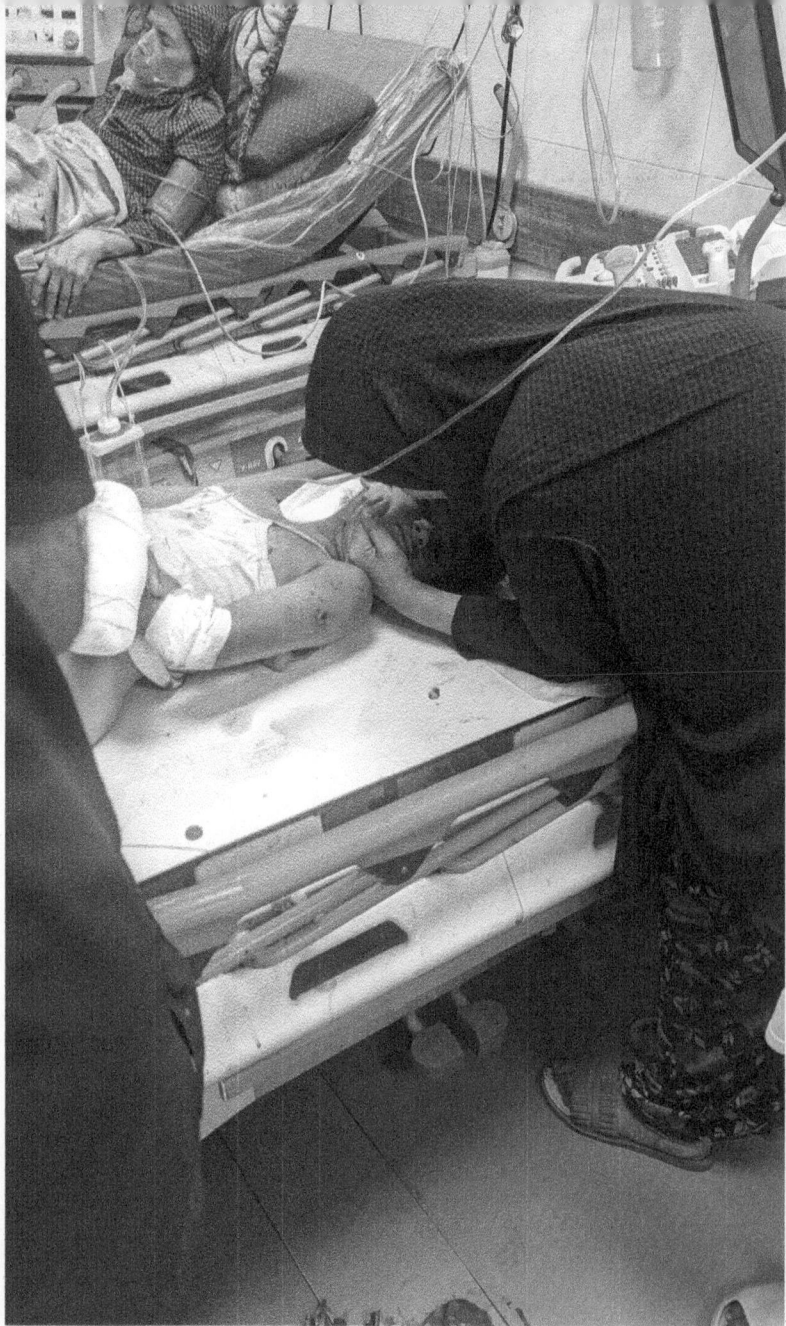

A mother comforting her daughter with severe blast injuries suffered while sleeping

Day 19
September 18 – This Feels Cruel

There were a few days last week where the mass casualties seemed to be less frequent. Today dispelled any notion I have that the end of the bombing is around the corner. The past 17 hours have been the busiest stretch of the trip so far. With the bombing of the tents outside the hospital, the daily bombings of Nuseirat and Bureij today, it's been non-stop. Today, it is impossible to see the end.

The main struggle yesterday was the lack of sterile gauze and other supplies that ground the ORs to a halt. We had several patients waiting most of the day in the ER, to either be transferred to a field hospital or for enough supplies to be scrounged from other hospitals nearby.

The mass casualties began arriving in the mid-afternoon. Several victims of explosive injuries arrived, two of whom were critical. The first was a 47-year-old woman with a catastrophic head injury who left a massive pool of blood on the floor. The other was ten-year-old Wajd, a young girl whose house was bombed, resulting in a gaping chest wound and abdominal bleeding. As part of our protocol, we had to completely remove all of her clothes to ensure there were no hidden injuries, which left Wajd laying on the stretcher in only her underwear. Because she was also losing blood, she was shivering uncontrollably, which we often see in shock. There are no blankets, sheets or even gowns at the hospital, so she lay there, shivering. The patient laying next to her, a 75-year-old woman with pneumonia, noticed us trying to find something to cover this girl and literally cut her blanket in half with a pair of scissors she borrowed from the nurse, so we could cover Wajd. A small moment of humanity carved out of a horrible scene.

After the ER seemed to be settled, Israar and I called it a night and around midnight I started my nightly writing. At around 1:30 am our phones lit up with a text from the senior overnight ER doctor that read "mass casualty." We raced down to the ER to find the entire team of ten overnight ER doctors hanging out on the front steps of the ER enjoying the night breeze and talking. I asked how they knew we would be receiving casualties and Dr. Wasim pointed to a nearby neighborhood and said, "The explosion was close." As soon as we started hearing the ambulance sirens in the distance, we all ran inside to prepare the ER for what was to come.

In total, five patients arrived simultaneously. All five were siblings sleeping in the tents near the hospital when a bomb landed near them. Several people were killed instantly and these children suffered severe injuries.

Eight-year-old Haysam and his 17-year-old brother Muhammad were brought to the Red Zone where they lay on the floor near each other, as their pools of blood inched closer. They were both awake and terrified, but 17-year-old Muhammad was trying to be strong and encourage his eight-year-old younger brother. While we pulled shrapnel from Muhammad's deep abdominal wounds and examined his leg fractures, he was calling his brother's name in between the moments of agony, letting Haysam know he was here with him.

Haysam had an open fracture of his left shin which was bleeding and dangling freely. We were unable to provide him with any pain medication as his leg was cleaned and manipulated. The brothers Haysam and Muhammad calling each other's names from across the floor in between screams of pain is something I don't think I'll ever be able to forget.

The three other siblings were on the floor of the waiting room. The most minor injury was an ankle fracture, but the other two sisters were in rough shape. Seven-year-old Warda had a clearly fractured skull, and her head was dented inwards and I could move the bones of her skull with my fingers. She was not responding and we bandaged her and sent her for a CT scan of her head to another hospital. I don't yet know how she fared, but I think she will end up having long-term brain damage if she survives.

Six-year-old Aseel broke me. This sweet girl, the age and size of my eldest daughter, was laying on the floor, shivering out of fear and pain. She broke the femur of her right leg, which is one of the most painful bones you can break in your body, and an injury that needs surgery. She also had a large and deep laceration next to her vagina, and her right index and middle fingers were blown off. Once she was stabilized, we brought her to the Red Zone, where the orthopedic surgeons began straightening her femur before the OR. She was staying composed the entire time until the painful parts, and a shortage of pain medications prevented us from sedating her for this procedure. While the surgeon was splinting her and straightening out her leg, she repeatedly screamed in Arabic "Oh my uncle, please be gentle!"

and then cried repeatedly for her mom. I've been careful not to share any pictures or videos of people in their worst moments as I feel like this dehumanizes them and we've all seen a year's worth of these videos anyways. But while the orthopedic surgeon was fixing this fracture and she was screaming for her mom I had to capture the moment briefly in audio, because I felt this moment needed to be shared and would resonate with anyone who would hear the cries of this terrified girl in pain. When her mom finally arrived, she buried her head into Aseel's face and kissed her repeatedly, while grabbing her head and comforting her with "Mama is here, Mama is here" until the procedure was complete.

On September 7th, the previous most difficult day of the trip, all the kids that died were sedated and didn't make a sound. There is a saying in emergency medicine that a quiet child is worse than a crying child (because the quiet child is likely sicker). But in its own way, hearing a child cry for their parent who isn't around to comfort them is one of the hardest aspects to accept and process in Gaza. Throughout my career, I don't think I can remember a single instance of a child crying in pain, or frightened, who didn't have a parent, close relative or loved one to comfort them. But in Gaza, this is a daily occurrence and it destroys me every single time. As a parent, your number one job is to protect your child. And when they're crying for you, you pick them up, kiss them and hug them tight until they slowly melt into your arms and shoulders, and you can feel their heartbeat slowing down (and this is when they're upset about something relatively trivial). That the children here very often don't get to be comforted like this while enduring grotesque and deforming injuries is incredibly difficult to think and write about.

We finally went to sleep around 5:30 am and planned to sleep until noon. At 10:30 am Israar and I were woken in a panic by our 16-year-old friend Bahajat, who lives in the hospital and helps the medical staff living here. In Arabic and speaking frantically, he said that his sister Elham was in the ER with a bomb injury and needed our help. We quickly changed and went downstairs to discover the ER waiting room floor covered with bodies from a mass casualty, due to yet another bombing at the Bureij displacement camp. Victoria was already in the emergency department and helping Elham with her facial wounds. Her eyes were swollen shut and she had multiple limb fractures. We sent her to another hospital for a CT scan and then to see an ophthalmologist. Later in the evening, we received the update that she has a right eye full of shrapnel, and the globe of her left eye had ruptured (her eyeball burst). Elham, a 30-year-old mother of small kids, is now totally blind and will never see her children again.

Laying on the floor next to her was 23-year-old Eman with a complete amputation of her left foot and a fracture of her right shin, where her foot was facing backwards. Her husband was hovering around us and waiting for us to stabilize her chest and abdominal wounds before we could get to her legs. You could tell he was desperate to see the extent of her leg injuries, and when we finally unwrapped her foot, he cried quietly with a look of anguish on his face, understanding his beloved wife would never be the same again.

This is the other part I haven't become numb to: That moment where family members see their loved ones in the

ER and the full extent of their injuries is revealed to them and you see that initial pain and heartbreak in their face. In the chaos of the resuscitation, you don't pay attention to it as there is simply too much to do. But once the dust settles, it hits you how many lives are affected by this tragedy. In time, I won't be able to remember all the injuries I've witnessed, but I will remember nearly every loved one's face and the scream of horror they make when they understand the reality of what befell their family. That cry stays with every doctor or nurse forever. Usually, its a handful of these moments that we remember, but in Gaza, this is a daily occurrence.

We took a short break and returned to the ER at 4 pm and were once again greeted with a similar scene as the morning: several injured bodies covering the floor of the ER, each in a pool of their own blood and surrounded by a massive crowd of media, family, other patients and gawkers. Chaos.

By 7 pm, a 15-year-old boy was dead from shrapnel wounds to his neck. Twenty-one-year-old Malik was declared brain dead after a massive quadcopter bullet both entered and exited his skull. A 20-year-old male needed to be rushed to the OR after rupturing his femoral artery and having his ankle blown off. There were several other critical injuries, including bleeding around the heart and chest, but its just too long of a list to write.

I've now mentioned three things that get me emotional. The fourth thing, when I have time to dwell on it, is the cruelty of all of this.

I promised I wouldn't editorialize or use controversial language and try to stay balanced. But how can I do this while staying true to my promise to report what I see with my own eyes? I'm not a scholar of war crimes, so I'll refrain from using these labels here. But I'm almost positive that if everyone I know witnessed this first hand, they would say that this is cruel. It *feels* cruel. It *feels* like torture, it *feels* unfair. It *feels* unjust. It *feels* … pointless. It feels like killing just for the sake of killing. Just go back and count how many children have been killed or maimed in my two weeks at a small hospital. Also remember that exactly half of the 2 million people in Gaza are children and any time you drop a bomb on an area, you have to assume that at least half of your victims will likely be children. How do you still drop a bomb after knowing this? Look at how many adults and sole providers for their families have been permanently disabled. How can we evaluate the psychological torture of dropping a bomb on a tent filled with sleeping children at 1 am?

I have often heard the saying "it's better to let a thousand guilty men go free than to punish one innocent man." I never really understood what this meant or the validity of it until I arrived here. I've seen too many *unquestionably* innocent children killed or deformed here to believe that any outcome is worth this. Malik's (the 20-year-old who was declared brain dead) father introduced himself to me so proudly: "I am his father" in the same way that I would look at my son when he first learned to stand up and glide on ice skates and say, "That's my boy." He was on a ventilator, brain dead, and waiting for death and his father still stood there beaming with pride at his son who he swears wasn't part of any resistance group. Who am I supposed to believe?

I was really hoping and praying that I would witness a ceasefire in my time here, but I've never felt more pessimistic about this than I do right now. As if to validate my feelings, it's now 2:30 am and a loud explosion just shook the windows I'm sitting beside. It was the kind of explosion that you feel in your chest. Now I have to decide if I should try to sleep or stay awake and listen for the sirens.

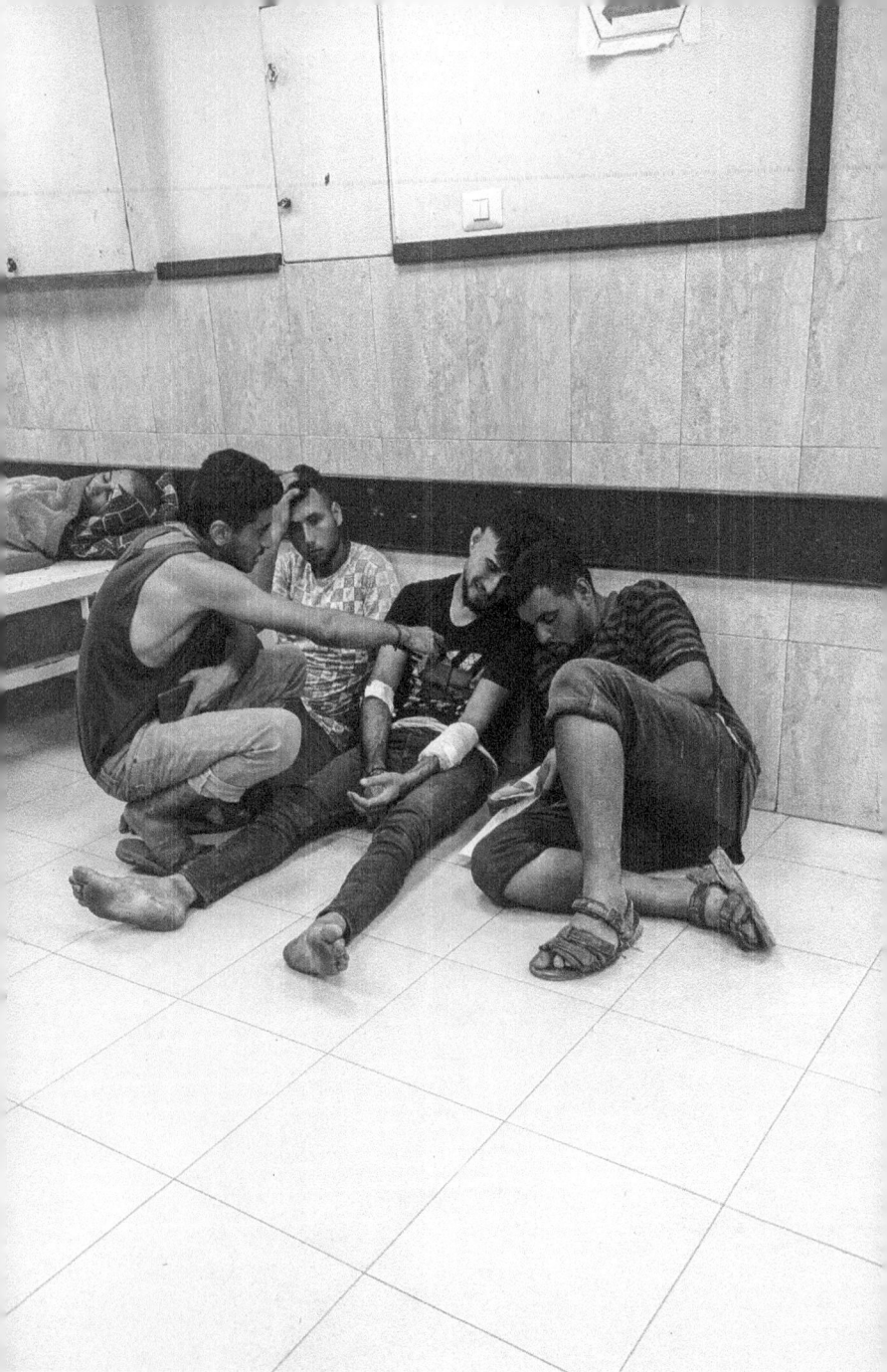

A man grieving the killing of his brother

Day 20
September 19 – Brothers

Part of our itinerary for today was a meeting with the Minister and Deputy Minister of Health at Al-Nasser Hospital to finalize plans to build the Humanity Auxilium Field Clinic in partnership with the MOH. This clinic will focus on providing much needed primary care services, given the complete collapse and lack of access to primary care in Gaza. The plans have already been created by our director of operations, Dr. Faiza Hussain, and CEO, Dr. Fozia Alvi, so this meeting was hopefully just to iron out any final details and answer questions to ensure Humanity Auxilium and the MOH are on the same page. The loud explosion at 2:30 am and another strong one at 5 am caused Israar and I to check the news, where we read reports of up to 80 people under the rubble in the Nuseirat again. Israar and I discussed it and decided it would be best to postpone the meeting and help in the ER, as this had the potential to be the largest MCI we've experienced on our mission. We went down to the ER at 9 am and not a single child patient arrived. We had no internet most of the day, so I don't actually know what happened to those people or if that number was even accurate. The physicians who read the same story said most of the people probably died.

It felt refreshing having a morning with no trauma patients and only sick medical cases.

There were two medical students in the ER this morning and I finally got the chance to offer them some teaching, like I had promised last week. The medical students in Gaza are all exceptionally bright and motivated. Their medical training has been on hold for the past year, and they have not received any classroom or didactic teaching during this time. Because of this, they crave any sort of teaching and it was very rewarding to spend a couple of hours with them.

My lack of sleep for the past 48 hours finally caught up with me and I ended up taking a three-hour nap this afternoon. It was one of those completely blackout naps where you wake up disoriented without setting an alarm.

After a quick bite, we went back down to the ER, for the evening and it was still very quiet. We did look after a sick three-year-old female with a congenital heart condition, a hypoplastic heart with one atrium and one ventricle, who was bleeding severely from her bowels and needed the ICU. At one point, her oxygen saturation dropped to 20 percent. The evening was super quiet, so the young doctors invited us to chill in their room and share in a falafel dinner that Dr. Saleh went across the street to find. The room is a small 10x15-ft room with small stretcher mattresses along the walls where ten or twelve of us sat and enjoyed each other's company, told stories and told jokes. After 15 years of ER work, I share with my junior ER colleagues that the excitement of inserting a breathing or chest tube or the adrenaline rush of caring for a critical patient is not what gives me or will give them satisfaction during the mid stages of their career. They're still vital skills, but the excitement of that eventually fades over time. What keeps me happy and fulfilled are the friendships I've made over the years. When

I'm driving to work on any given morning, evening or night, what I'm excited about is to spend time and catch up with my friends. This is what I felt sitting in that small room sharing a meal with my new friends. They shared that they felt the same way, in that they are here out of a sense of duty to their people, but they are fulfilled by spending time with their friends and the comradery of the ER. Sitting with these amazing doctors in that moment, I didn't miss Canada and truly felt like I was home.

At 9:30 pm, a familiar commotion filled the ER waiting room, so we jumped to our feet and ran to the Red Zone. What we saw was a young man in his 20s laying on the floor, covered in blood. I started to get to work by cutting off his shirt and pants to find the source of the bleeding: a gaping wound to his left chest directly over his heart. It was only then that I actually looked at him to see that his face was completely pale and his pupils were fixed and dilated. He was already dead. I performed a cardiac ultrasound to confirm what I and all the doctors and nurses in the room already knew, pronounced him dead and then stepped aside to allow his brother to lay beside him on the floor and grieve. Many of the 15 doctors and nurses in the room stood there and watched his brother cry, grab his dead brother's face, hug him, kiss his bloody face and chest, stroke his beard and scream at him not to leave.

I stood in the corner of the room trying to absorb the moment and thought of my own brother, who is five years older than me. Growing up, he's always been the person I spent the most time with playing and watching sports, video games, and even fighting with. I've always looked up to him, and as the older brother to a skinny kid, he's always had a protective instinct towards me, even when we lived together when I was a medical student and he was a resident in Ottawa. We've managed to stay close in our adult years through our love of NFL football, often meeting every Sunday to spend the day watching games together (at least before I had kids). As we've gotten older, I feel like I'm strangely becoming more protective of him now, and I think this comes from a long-standing worry about not having him in my life. Watching this young man grieve over his brother's shockingly sudden passing brought these feelings to the surface for me, and just as I wrote yesterday, this is just another scream to add to the list of those I won't forget.

After about 15 minutes, his body was moved to another area. As soon as he left the room, the Red Zone instantly filled with three more trauma victims who were suddenly placed on the floor in front of us, all of whom were males in their 20s. Upon examination, two of these young men were immediately pronounced dead on arrival. They remained on the floor as we tried to revive the only living victim, and it was difficult not to trip over the dead bodies around us while we worked. This man had wounds that shattered both of his legs and had lost at least two to three liters of blood and was in clinical shock. We filled him with blood and he was rushed to the operating room. When it was all over, I just stood there with blood all over my arms blankly staring into space trying to process what just happened. I thought that by writing these journals, I would instantly gain perspective by taking the time to reflect, but I'm slowly realizing that only when I'm back home and separated from the chaos will I be able to gain any clarity from all of this.

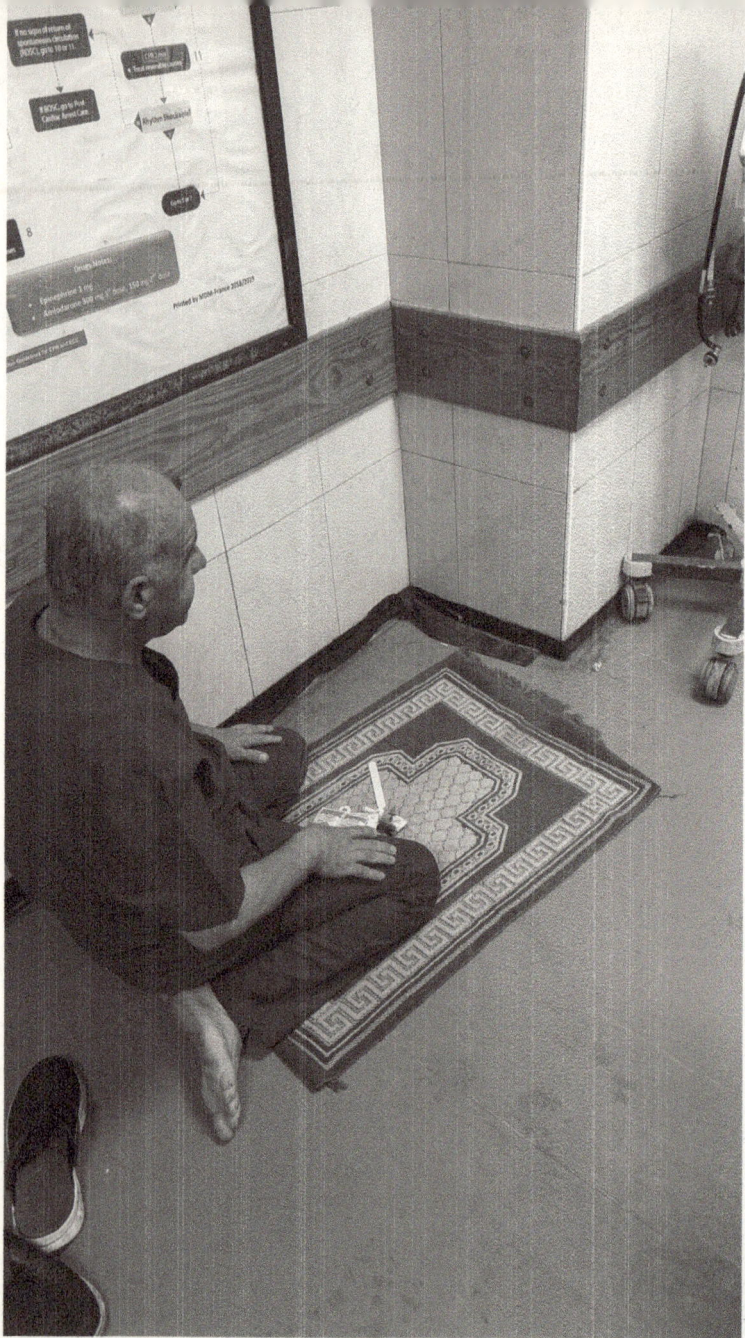

A nurse praying in the emergency department between mass casualty incidents

Day 21
September 20 – Compassion

My original intention for writing in this journal was for it to act as an outlet and a therapeutic space for me to help process the heavy events each day, but today feels different. I've been sharing my reflection with friends and well-wishers but have been asked to stop due to some unknowable and invisible security concern that might place at risk our team's ability to safely exit Gaza in twelve days. I've enjoyed sharing my thoughts with people so that my moments of grief, anger, frustration and reflection could be shared by others and in doing so, my feelings would hopefully become their feelings and I wouldn't have to carry these emotions alone. I've been encouraged to continue writing but today, it feels like my words are just being lost in the vacuum of space. Writing in this journal today feels lonely. You know that feeling of traveling together with a person or group and then that person leaves and you think, "Well that just sucked the fun out of this." That's what this feels like right now.

My secondary reason for sharing real-time thoughts was the hope to bring the plight of these people to the front and center of everyone's consciousness back home. Knowing my own short attention span, I worry that (a) no one will even bother to read any of this after I return and (b) no one will even care because it's old news.

Perhaps I have been delusional in the first place to think that anything I write would be able to move people's hearts or mobilize people. I have to accept, as I always should have, that my responsibility is simply to do the work entrusted to me and it's only The Most High who can turn hearts and minds.

Today we arrived in the ER and there was "only" one trauma patient, who we followed throughout the entire day. We spent some time in Dr. Haddad's office where we happily shared with him that Humanity Auxilium is funding the tent that will serve as the new Yellow Zone for his department. Being the medical director of my emergency department at my hospital back home, I'm just as excited and invested in Dr. Haddad's need for a tent to help offload ER congestion. Just as my department in Canada often combats congestion issues, so does his. The only difference is that his department is half the size and sees five times the patient volume. His plan is to take all of the patients that are congesting the hallways of the current Yellow Zone, and move them to the outside of the hospital with a large spacious tent. This will allow the doctors to offer better care for the sickest and most high-risk patients in the ER. Dr. Haddad is constantly motivated by ER flow and patient quality, which is something I relate to.

While having this conversation in his office, there was a loud fracas in the waiting room, and we peeked our heads outside to see a scrum involving around 10–15 people. At the center were the family members of two patients, with the crowd trying to separate them. It lasted about a minute, which felt like an eternity as it's happening, but fortunately no one was injured before they were escorted out of the ER and business carried on as though nothing happened.

Going back to the trauma patients, this was eight-year-old Yazan, a young boy who suffered a catastrophic head injury in an explosion, and had exposed brain matter and was declared a "hopeless" case, which we would classify as "palliative" or "comfort care" in Canada. He had several other injuries including multiple sites of shrapnel in his lungs and his abdomen that we monitored carefully. Despite him being palliative, multiple doctors from various specialties came down to offer care to his various wounds. One specific moment that moved me was the care and compassion the surgical team showed when carefully suturing his multiple facial lacerations. Despite the throngs of patients in the hospital and multiple demands on their time, it was still important for them to perform an excellent cosmetic closure to Yazan's face, even though he will likely die before his cuts heal. They would be forgiven if they said this was a pointless exercise, but they still wanted to offer this child and his parents the compassion the bombs didn't give them as they waited for death. I thought this was beautiful.

Because of the low number of traumas today, Yazan actually spent more than 14 hours in a Red Zone bed, which I haven't witnessed yet. His family was by his side all day and his mom often fixed his hair, periodically wiped his bleeding nose, and adjusted his blanket to ensure his feet weren't exposed. All the while, both parents just stood beside his bed because there are no chairs, and stared at their dying son with a quiet dignity, but pained expressions on their faces. At one point, we rolled him onto his side to examine his chest wounds and changed his dressings. This

111

is when we realized that he wasn't even laying on a mattress. He was laying on a hard wooden/composite material of the stretcher and his parents brought in a small piece of cardboard to place under his buttocks and back to soften things for him. This dying child could not even get something soft to lay on. It was 1 am when we finally called it a night, but he was still in the ER, waiting for a bed upstairs.

Earlier in the day I went outside for some fresh air and heard something I had not yet heard before … gunfire. It was multiple shots, not too far away, and I didn't think much of it. But shortly after, an 18-year-old woman arrived in the ER with a gunshot wound to the left chest. The bullet entered near her collarbone and stopped in the middle of her left chest very near her heart. The staff studied the wound and concluded that she was shot by a bullet that was intended to be shot in the air, but still had enough force because of a low trajectory to hit her based on the location and size of the entry wound. She received a chest tube and will hopefully recover.

The final rush of the night arrived at 9:30 pm, after a bombing at the Nuseirat camp. A 13/14-year-old male had a serious fracture and possible vascular injury of his right leg. Next to him on the floor of the waiting room lay a 20-year-old female who appeared half her age because of her cerebral palsy, evident by the flexed and rigid posture of her limbs and facial features. She too had compound fractures of her right leg, but the most concerning injury was the blood pouring from her left eye. I wasn't able to follow up with her, but I'm concerned that she has lost the vision in her left eye from either embedded shrapnel or a ruptured globe.

The night ended with a man in his late 60s being rushed to a Red Zone in cardiac arrest. We worked on him for several minutes but could not regain his pulse and we pronounced him dead at just past midnight.

It's crazy to think about but I'm heading to sleep feeling like today was a good day. But if you're keeping score, here it is: an eight-year-old is brain dead after an explosion and about to die. An elderly man is dead after waiting in the waiting room for two hours. An 18-year-old woman was shot in the chest and a 20-year-old disabled woman is now partially blind. This is what I now consider a good day in Gaza.

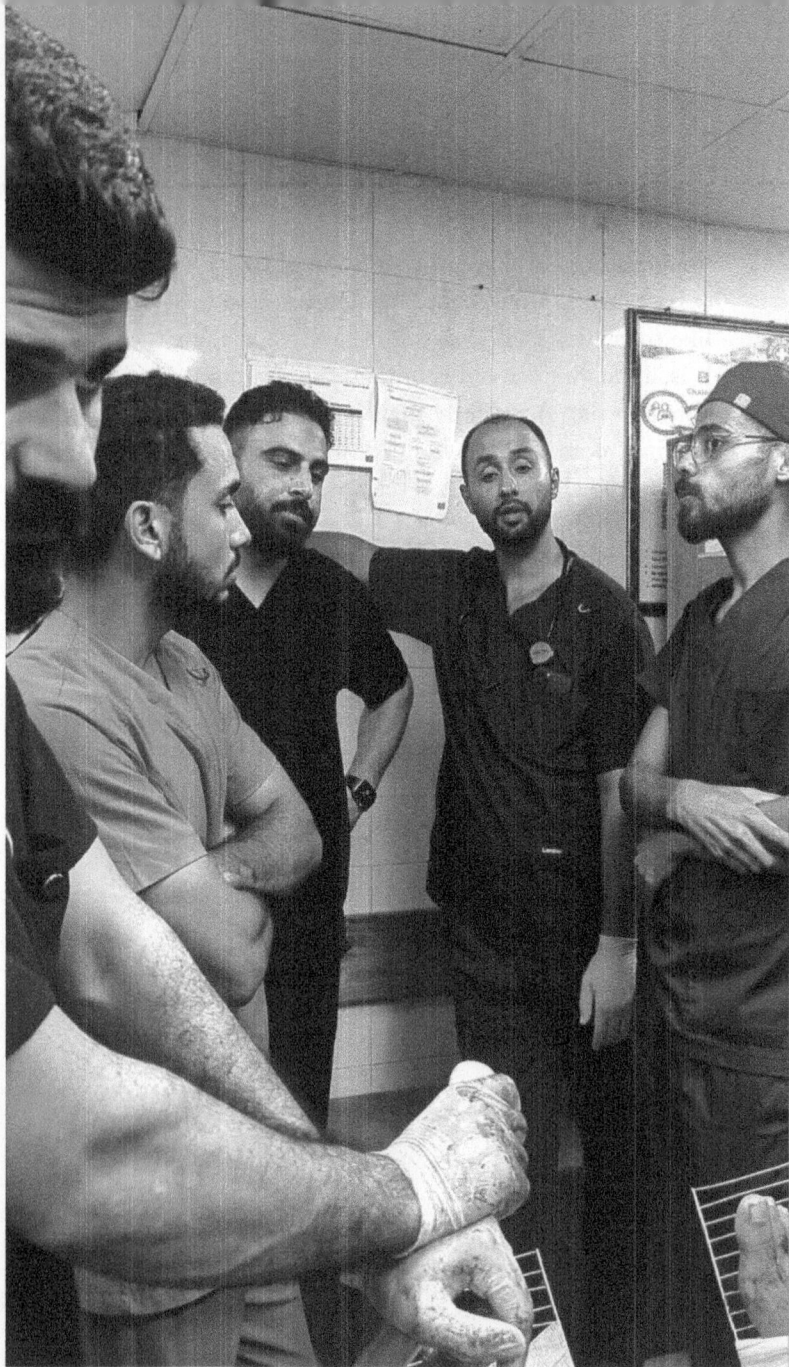

Physicians discussing trauma patients for the operating room

Day 22
September 21 – Hopeful Case

Today, I was able to offer something I never thought I'd be able to in my first three weeks at the Al Aqsa Hospital. I wrote earlier about caring deeply about providing excellent end-of-life care for my patients back home and this is something that has been nearly impossible in overcrowded resuscitation rooms with patients laying on the floor. Today was different.

In the afternoon, a 74-year-old woman was wheeled into the Red Zone, appearing pale and taking sporadic, gasping breaths. We immediately jumped on her stretcher and began chest compressions, and began advanced cardiac life support (ACLS). After 30 minutes, we regained a pulse and she was semi-conscious, but it appeared that her heart might still stop at any moment, and we would finally have to cease our efforts.

At this moment, we invited her children to join her at the head of the bed and talk to her, encouraging them to tell their mom everything that was in their heart, in case she was to die. They all lined up and it was a beautiful moment to witness them kissing their mom's hands, face and head, and honoring her through their tears and words. Although heartbreaking, it was still a beautiful thing to witness this family saying a potential final farewell to their beloved mother. Death has been so sudden here that I haven't really observed any final goodbyes like this. Over time, I've learned that this part of the care we provide to patients is the one that families are most thankful for.

But then something amazing happened: after another 30 minutes, her heart started contracting stronger, her breathing improved and she started waking up and even talking. Even in Canada, I wouldn't have expected this elderly patient with a very sick heart to live. That she was able to recover and be admitted to the Cardiac Care Unit was incredible. It reaffirmed my belief that we are entrusted to do the work with the skills we've been blessed with, but that life and death are ultimately not in our hands.

Around 8 pm, 40-year-old Shahdi arrived with rapidly deteriorating consciousness and was placed on the floor of the Red Zone. He was walking after dinner and was struck by a bullet. It hit him in the back of the head, exploding his skull and leaking a large amount of brain on the floor. Normally, I've seen this quickly declared a "hopeless" case, but when the neurosurgeon examined him, he said if we could act quickly and insert a breathing tube and get a CT, he might be able to operate on him to relieve some of the pressure. It still took a couple of hours because the broken CT scanner at Al Aqsa meant we had to transfer him to another hospital for a CT. When it was finally complete, several of us, including Shahdi's family, grouped in front of a computer screen and eagerly listened to the neurosurgeon's opinion. "Let's operate and give him a chance."

Even if it's all you can offer, a little bit of hope can sometimes make all the difference.

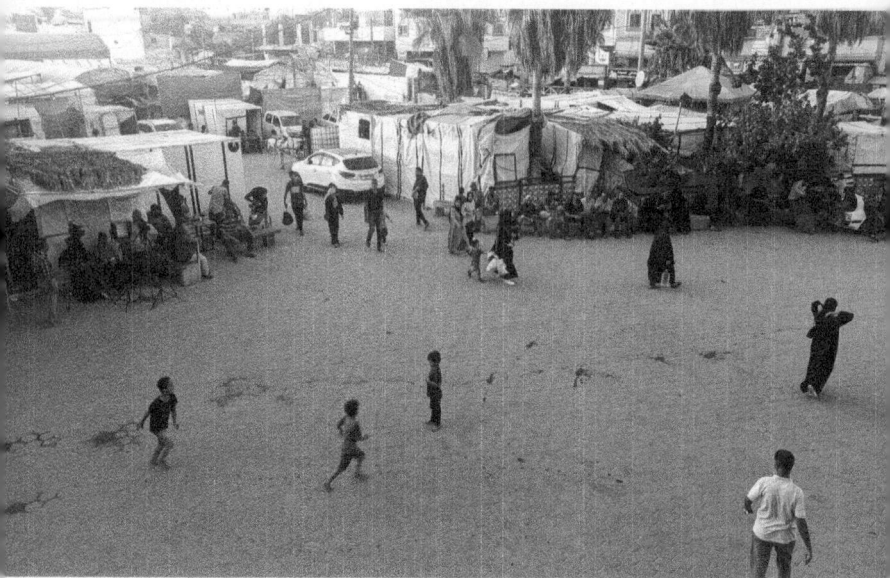

Children playing in the courtyard of Al Aqsa Hospital

Day 23
September 22 – I Miss Everything

A couple of updates: Our four-year-old friend Yusuf with the lung contusions still has a breathing tube and is in the Intensive Care Unit. It's been two weeks and he's failed multiple attempts to remove this breathing tube, as he goes into respiratory failure shortly after. He otherwise looks amazing and his scalp wounds are healing well, but his lungs have been slow to recover. He's scheduled for a tracheostomy (a tube inserted into his throat) today or tomorrow, but they're waiting to find the right size tube for him. We try to visit him every day and when we can't, we usually run into his father in the courtyard of the hospital, who happily greets us and shares updates.

The patient who Victoria is trying to medevac is now on the list, but is still waiting on various levels of administrative clearance. There is a hospital in Jordan ready to take her and the funds are available through Humanity Auxilium, and it is now only a matter of getting the MOH and COGAT to agree to mobilize. Her wounds are improving, but for her future quality of life, she needs a reconstructive surgery that can't occur in Gaza.

Yesterday was a quiet day in the emergency department, with only a few non-critical trauma patients. In the late evening hours, we spent time talking with the resuscitation nurses in the empty Red Zone and shared stories, some happy and some sad. For the past three weeks I've been working with an experienced and excellent nurse named Shahdi, a 31-year-old man, who is very soft spoken and doesn't joke around as much as some of the other nurses. Once I learned what happened to him, I understood why.

Shahdi was living and working in Gaza City, where he lived with his wife of seven years Samah and their two sons: six-year-old Essam and five-year-old Ammar. He continued to work at Al-Shifa Hospital in Gaza City in the early days of the conflict because they hadn't been giving any instruction to relocate. Samah was also eight months pregnant with their third child, and they intended to stay in their home and close to extended family for as long as they believed it was safe. And besides, they've lived through other sieges and have been relatively unscathed, so why would this time be any different?

Anyone who's had a baby on the way can relate to the mix of excitement and vulnerability you feel in the weeks and months leading up to the due date. You're hopeful, but also know that anything can happen to mom or baby during the remaining days of pregnancy and even labor, and very little is in your control. Whether you know if it's a boy or a girl, you start daydreaming about ... well ... everything. First foods, first words, first steps, first day of school, playing games and sports, making blanket forts, graduations, weddings and even as far as becoming grandparents yourself. If you're lucky to have good health and security, it can be one of the happiest times in your life.

As the sun was setting on a day last fall, Shahdi was working an evening shift at Al-Shifa when he got a call from a friend that his mother-in-law was looking for him urgently. When he finally saw her, she was in the ER and he knew something terrible had happened. She told them that a missile hit the neighbor's house but the force of impact had collapsed the room where Samah and Essam were sitting. Ammar was in the next room and was okay. When Shahdi finally found Samah and Essam in the ER, they were both in critical condition. Ammar was struck in the head with shrapnel and had a serious head injury. Samah was in even worse condition as she had a serious abdominal and diaphragmatic injury with internal bleeding. Shahdi remembers trying to help, but his colleagues forced him to be a husband and not a nurse, so he stayed by his wife's side while his mother-in-law stayed with Essam.

Samah was rushed to the operating room where she had an emergency caesarean section to deliver their baby. Despite their quick action, their baby had died from the impact. It was a boy and they named him Samir after Samah's grandfather. After the surgery to repair Samah's abdominal injuries, she was transferred to the ICU where she lived only for another 30 minutes, dying with Shahdi by her side. He buried Samah and Samir the following day at noon, mom and baby sharing a grave in a cemetery in Gaza City.

For the following 35 days, Essam and Ammar accompanied their father to work because there is no such thing as bereavement leave in Gaza and the hospital (he mistakenly thought) was the only place he could guarantee their safety. It took some time, but Essam has mostly recovered from his injuries with only minimal motor deficits. Shahdi shared that their kids miss their mom's presence every day, and when asked what the children know about her and their baby brother they say, "Mama is in heaven, waiting for us." I asked him what he misses the most about Samah and he smiled and said, "everything." He still has not visited Samah's resting place since the day he placed her in the earth, because the area isn't safe and he was forced to relocate after the first siege of Al-Shifa to find new work in a safer location. He is hopeful that he can visit them as soon as the bombs stop.

Shahdi wasn't especially eager to share his personal tragedy as some of the other nurses in the room. Even some of the nurses who've known him for the past few months were surprised to know that he was carrying this burden and loss with him. He wasn't excitedly telling me "go tell the world my story!" He simply said "everyone in Gaza has lost someone close, and my story isn't special." He appeared like someone who despite his heartache had accepted his share of the events surrounding him. He looked like someone missing his best friend.

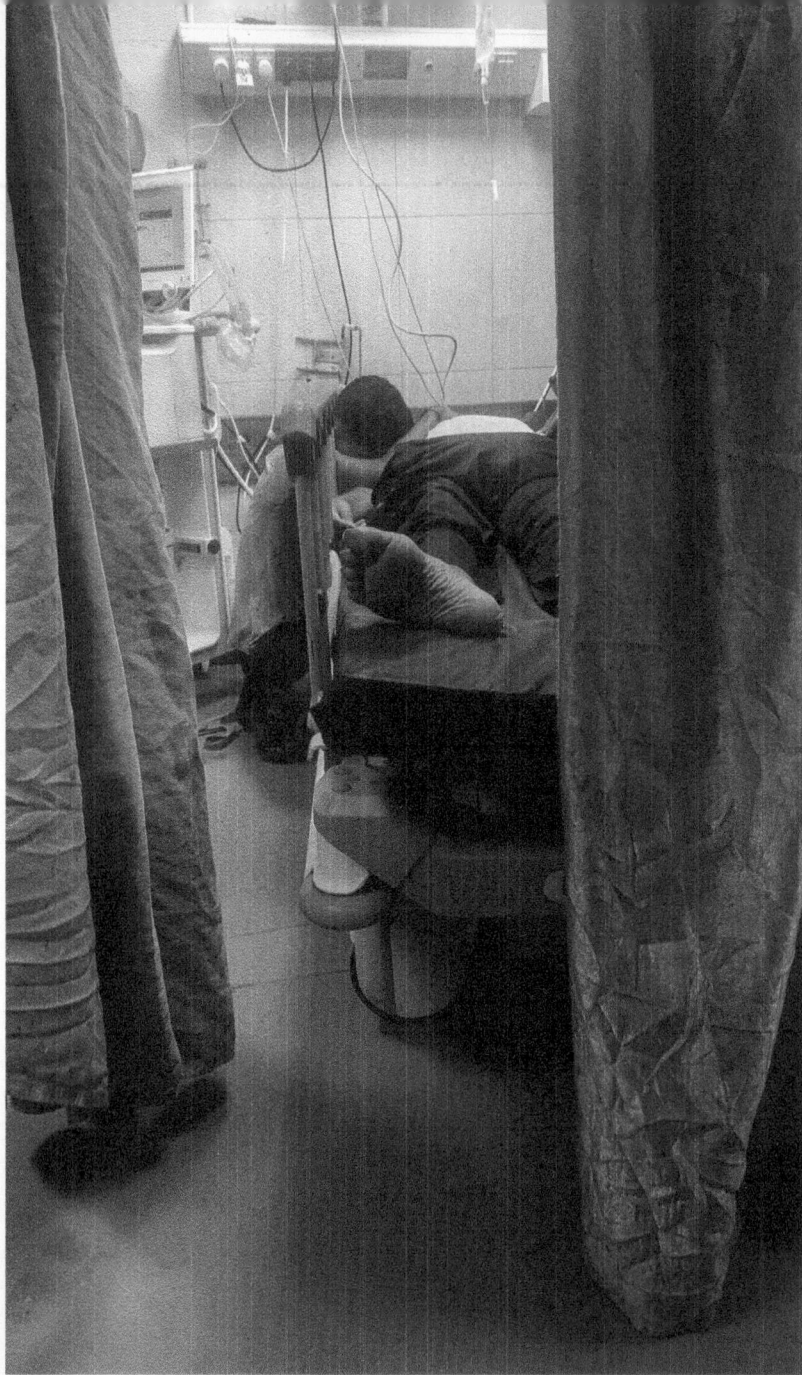

A young man grieving his deceased father

Day 24
September 23 – A Day of Death

After a quiet day yesterday, today was the opposite. It was a day filled with death. A lot of death. It felt like we spent the day just watching people die. Another 4 am bombing of the Nuseirat camp brought mass casualties to our door. When we arrived in the late morning, there were multiple people scattered all over the waiting room floor as has become the daily routine of the Al Aqsa Hospital.

The first people to catch my attention were a family of four, a father and his three children laying in his lap or near him. The father was sitting against a wall with his right ear completely ripped apart and oozing blood. A seven- and a twelve-year-old boy sat near him and with lacerations and leg injuries but they appeared stable. The most injured family member was eight-year-old Anas, who was laying on the floor, semi-conscious with a depressed skull fracture and blood and air in his brain. His face and eyes were swollen shut and he had an arterial injury in his right wrist that was awaiting an immediate repair in the OR.

In the resuscitation room, a 26-year-old man had suffered a right below knee amputation when his leg was blown off and he was waiting to be transferred to another hospital because our operating room lacked sterile surgical gowns and gauze. Despite our best attempts to sedate him and keep him comfortable, his moans filled the Red Zone for most of the morning and afternoon.

Next to him was a 61-year-old female named Najah, who had a serious head injury, who died in the early afternoon. Next to her was 17-year-old Asser, who also required monitoring for a head injury.

Around 1:30 pm, we received another wave of casualties from an airstrike at Al-Shati camp.

The first to arrive was a 43-year-old man with a compound fracture of his right shin and shrapnel injuries that were soaking his pants with blood. The second was a young man in his 20s. I'm running out of ways to describe these injuries, but the best way that I can illustrate it is that this man appeared shredded. He had so many wide and gaping wounds to his chest, abdomen and extremities that it looked like someone had just taken a giant, flaming hot grater to him. His legs were broken in so many pieces that his shins bent the way his knees normally would, and he was covered in dirt, burns, shrapnel and blood and his head was smashed in. Within minutes of his arrival, it was apparent that there was no chance of reviving him, and we pronounced him dead. With no family present to grieve him, we moved fast to remove him from the room.

During this wave and even the morning wave, there were at least four people that were brought to the Red Zone who were either dead or taking their final breaths. It all happened so fast that in 30 seconds, a couple of doctors would quickly examine the patient and either pronounce them dead or declare that they can't be saved. Sometimes they would move a dead patient in and out of the room so quickly that I didn't even look up from what I was doing to notice that they had just declared someone dead. When they're brought into the Red Zone in a panic, it is often on a sheet carried by people at the four corners and not even on a stretcher, placed on the floor, and then removed just as fast. The ages of the people that we pronounced dead today ranged from their 20s to their 50s. We also saw people that were trapped under the rubble for hours, including a 25-year-old man with obvious penetrating and crush injuries to his neck and his entire body whom we declared dead on arrival. Usually, most of these patients don't even make it to the hospital or are pronounced dead in the waiting room, but more patients than usual made it to the resuscitation room today. Eventually, things settled for a few hours because, well, most people were dead, which gave us a chance to take a breather and catch up with the staff.

Probably the toughest case of the evening was a 61-year-old male who was severely short of breath from uncertain diagnosis. Our portable emergency department ultrasound machine stopped working a few days ago and there is no one who can repair it. The same goes for CT, which has been broken for the past six months and there is no chance of repair in sight because the necessary equipment and personnel is not being allowed into Gaza. There's also no portable chest X-ray, which is a mobile machine that can perform an X-ray at the bedside. The most difficult aspect of providing care was being forced to wait over an hour for someone to find an oxygen tank to take him to the X-ray department. This oxygen tank never arrived while he continued to deteriorate, and we lacked an ability to make a convincing diagnosis. During the two hours we cared for him, we tried our best with what we had, but it became clear that he was rapidly deteriorating and would likely die.

We kept his four sons informed throughout the process, but you could see their faces start to change from confident to concerned and then finally to grief as they understood that he couldn't be saved. But it's only after the staff begin saying, "*Allah Yarham,*" which means "May God have mercy on him," as an informal declaration of death, that it really hits the family.

And there's nothing really that can prepare you for that moment. His sons gathered towards their dead father and kissed his hands and face while his youngest son knelt beside his father and quietly wept.

I have to be honest that it was frustrating. Two hours, feeling that I was just watching helplessly as a man slowly and uncomfortably died without doing what I came here to do, lacking the tools I felt I needed. My experience back home has taught me that even if I had the most advanced modern medical technology at my disposal, we still see patients die despite our best efforts. This patient once again reminded me that life and death don't belong to us and I have to accept that it was "his appointed time."

After several minutes, I went back and offered my condolences in broken Arabic to one of his sons. His son hugged me and placed his arm around my shoulders and when I said, "*ana asif,*" which means "I'm sorry," he placed his hand on top of his head and then mine, which is a traditional way of saying that he accepts and greatly appreciates what we did. It was still reassuring to know that despite their heartbreak, they understood that we tried our best. And it was just as important for me to let them know that we tried our best.

Before I could call it a night and start writing, I saw eight-year-old Anas in the hallway. He had his surgery and his head was wrapped but he still appeared a bit restless and irritable. It was around 11 pm and his mom was standing beside him, fanning him with a piece of cardboard for hours. He likely will be admitted for several days and I need to be hopeful that he can recover.

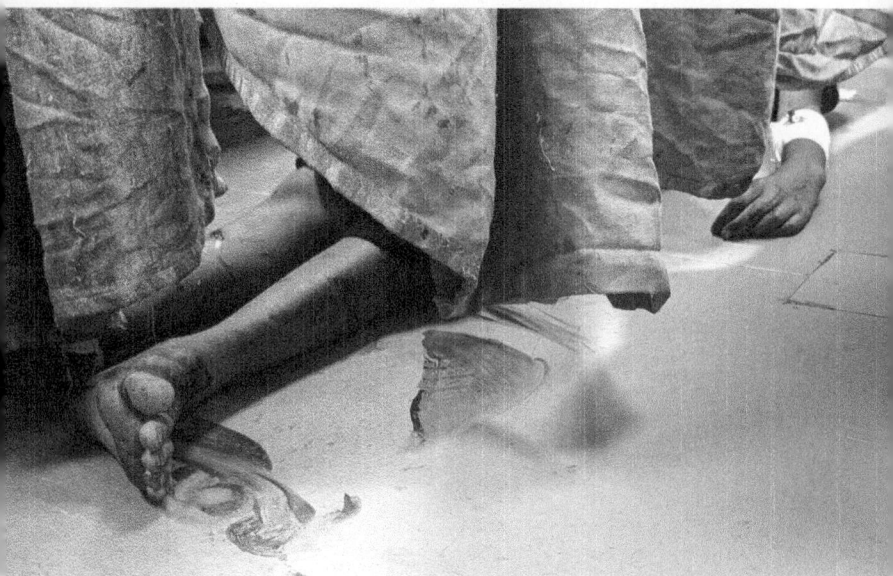

A dying child lays on the floor for hours

Day 25
September 24 – Nameless Faces

I don't remember any of their names. There were too many to keep track of. I lost count. I made an effort to note names to try to learn about who patients are as people, but today was impossible. It was wave after wave after wave. For the third or fourth time since I've been here, I'm beginning a journal with "today was the worst day." After three weeks, I thought I had experienced a large enough sample size to know how bad it could get. But today proved my assumptions wrong again. Nuseirat was hit several times today and Bureij was the first. Even as I went to the front steps of the ER to catch my breath, we could hear the gunfire from the Apache helicopters flying overhead, causing terror down below.

When we started at noon, the first wave of casualties just arrived and we got acclimated and began our work. We were fortunate that Victoria decided to join us for a day in the emergency department, and her presence couldn't have been timed any better. It would be exhausting to list all the patients we were involved with today, so I'll give a quick summary.

Of the patients with critical, life-threatening and catastrophic injuries today, half were children. Innocent children. Harmless little humans who are described as "collateral damage." I can't imagine a more dehumanizing word than "collateral damage." I hate this expression so much. What an abhorrent way to describe a human life.

We treated a four-year-old girl with a massive bleed in her chest; I currently don't know whether she is alive or dead.

We treated a three-year-old boy with severe head injuries and brain bleeding.

We treated an eleven-year-old boy who is now brain dead from yet another catastrophic brain injury and exposed brain matter.

We cared for a ten-year-old girl with extensive tissue loss to her left leg and severe internal abdominal bleeding; I also don't know if she is currently alive or dead.

We tended to a 16-year-old boy with shredded intestines and abdominal organs.

We also looked after multiple young adults in their 20s, 30s and 40s with head injuries and exposed brain matter, now just waiting to die.

This is not even half my list. Just when we thought we had things sort of under control, a fresh pile of bodies was dropped to the Red Zone floor with a crowd of more than 20 people trying to figure out who had the most immediately life-threatening injuries in all the chaos.

By the time we ended our shift, two children and five adults were either brain dead or dying. Several other children and young adults are in the operating room or being observed, and I don't know if they lived or died. This doesn't include the several patients who were pronounced dead in the ER waiting room upon arrival. I also saw a man who was completely eviscerated. And I don't mean it figuratively, but with his actual intestines hanging outside of his body.

I mentioned previously that every day in the ER has a theme. And the theme of today was that nearly every adult or child who was unconscious (whatever the cause) vomited all over themselves. Their last meals poured slowly from their mouths and nostrils all over their face, down their neck and chest, leaving them with their head lying in a pool of their vomit and blood. Most of the children we treated today were not accompanied by any loved ones, so they often sat with their head, neck and clothes covered in vomit for sometimes more than an hour. Normally, these patients would have been cleaned immediately, but it often took some time to finally clean them, due to the exhaustive wave of patients arriving in the emergency department. At one point, Victoria had to grab a semi-conscious three-year-old boy to prevent him from rolling over into a pile of his own vomit and blood. And even when we did finally clean them, we still had children with their hair crusted with dried vomit. Just a nightmare of sights and smells to witness.

Talking to most of the staff, they didn't even seem particularly fazed by all of this. They actually told me that today was barely 30 percent of what they were experiencing just a few months ago. I've been at this pace for three weeks, and I'm starting to feel my body physically wearing down, so I can't imagine what my colleagues who have been working at this pace, with this stress and limited resources for an entire year must be feeling. I don't have to worry about searching for water or food. I don't have the mental burden of worrying about my family's safety. They're so clearly exhausted and burnt out, but they continue to try their best. I came here in the hopes of offering the staff some small respite, but today feels no different, if not worse, than on September 3.

I'm sitting here at the end of the day wondering how it was allowed to get to this point. All I want is for their nightmare to end.

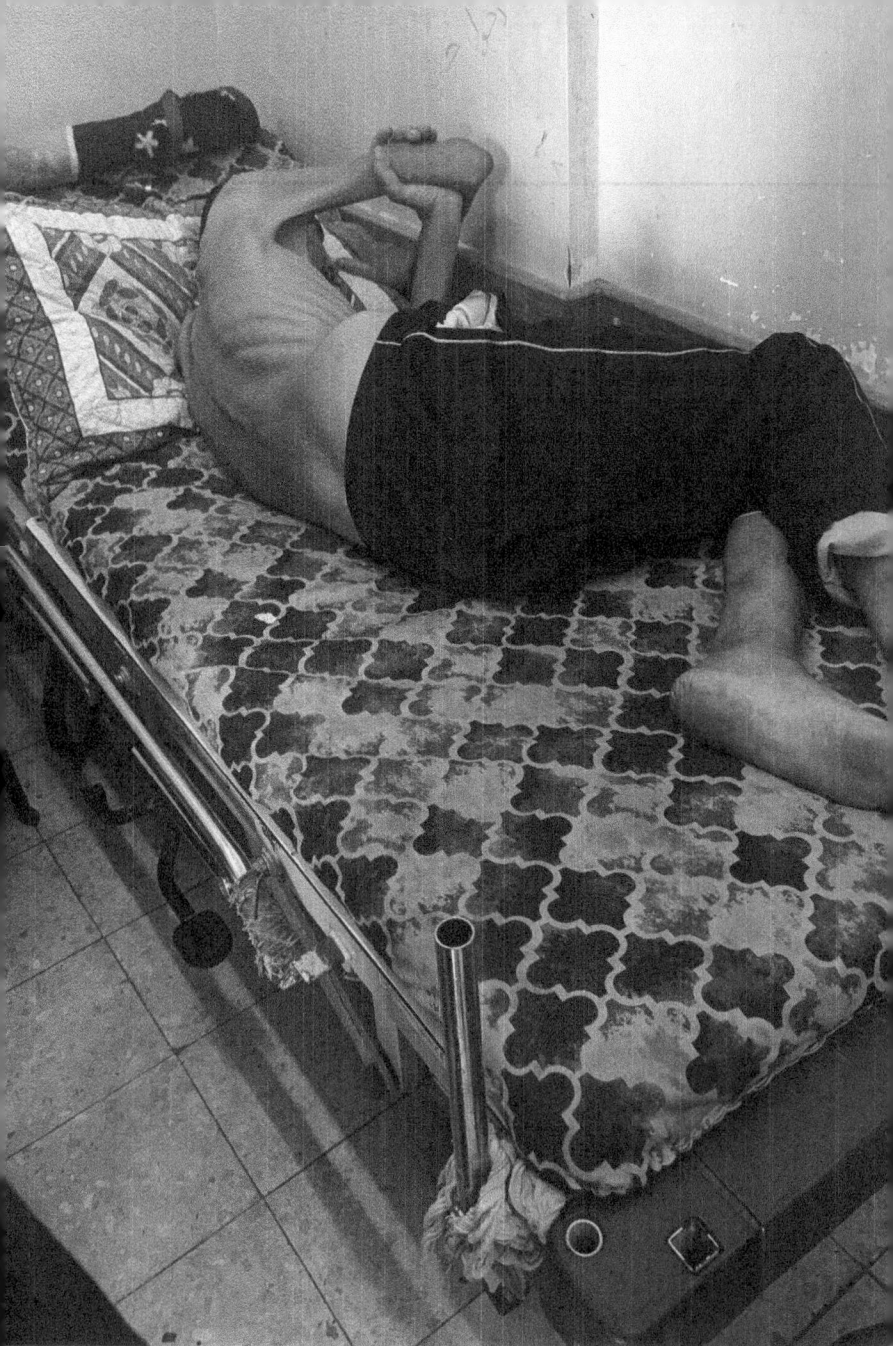

One of many severely malnourished patients
on the surgical floor of Al Aqsa Hospital

Day 26
September 25 – Surgery Rounds

Yusuf update: He has received his tracheostomy and no longer requires sedation. His eyes are open and he is beginning to eat. His hands are no longer tied like they were when he was pulling at his tube in the past two weeks. It's simultaneously hilarious and heartbreaking that even with his hands tied, he somehow managed to lean onto his side and pull out his breathing tube five times in a single day! It fills me with happiness to see his father every day. While he's sitting on a curb in the courtyard, he will notice us and jump up with a warm smile and greeting. I still remember the anger, grief and frustration he displayed when we first met while we were performing CPR on his son. To see him smiling and happy and hopeful is incredibly heartwarming.

I followed Victoria and the surgery team today for their rounds to better understand what happens after many of these patients head to the operating room. Dr. Haysam was the staff surgeon working alongside her. There are a few themes that I observed:

1. There are *so* many patients who have bed sores. I'm not talking about small bed stores. These are massive craters that have eroded from their superficial buttocks deep into their pelvis. The main reason that this has occurred is that the hospital is nearly three times over capacity so nurses

137

don't have the time to use pillows and shift weight several times a day. This leaves patients suffering from strokes, Parkinson's, paraplegia, and other injuries laying still for several hours with pressure in one spot. Some of the bed sores that I've seen look beyond repair and will likely eventually lead to patients dying.

2. There are patients *everywhere* in the hospital. Rooms are full. Patients are laying on small mattresses they brought from home in hallways, stairwells, lobbies, outside administrative offices … pretty much anywhere there is open floor space. Yesterday, I saw a man hammering 2x4s of wood into the hospital walls and ceiling in a corner of a hallway, creating a cubic-like structure that he was likely going to call home for the foreseeable future. Just outside of the room where I sleep a three-year-old girl has been on a stretcher for the entirety of our stay.

3. There are *so* many amputees, both children and adults. I've never seen as many amputees in my entire career as I've seen in a single day. It's something I noticed on my first days here, but became part of the background over the past four weeks. Walking the hallways at Al Aqsa Hospital, you'll also see countless patients in beds with external fixators which are devices used to repair fractures. One of the reasons they choose this method as opposed to the internal fixation I'm accustomed to is that the wounds are often dirty, and the risk of infection is very high if you close the skin. If you haven't seen a picture of an external fixator, do a quick internet search and you'll see what I'm talking about.

4. While walking through the sea of people on my way to the ER, I've often smelt what appears to be rotting, necrotic

or infected flesh. I didn't see any of these wounds today, but Victoria described that many of her patients have actually done quite well postoperatively but several others have such complicated penetrating injuries that their wounds have become infected and each day she sees them worsening. In some cases, she's seen them improve, but in a few others, she has seen them decline towards what is likely their gradual and painful death. There are many determinants to successful wound healing, including clean gauze that can be changed daily, a hygienic environment, close monitoring, antibiotics and proper nutrition. Very often, these determinants aren't met, causing a worsening of these postoperative complications that were easily preventable.

5. I've observed so many obviously malnourished and cachectic patients today on rounds. I think today was the first day that I really noticed how skinny and wasted many of these patients appear. Usually, in the emergency department, I see kids that appear to be three to four years younger than their actual age. It was unnerving to be able to easily count ribs and vertebrae of adults who would have been much heavier and healthier one year ago. Walking the halls on rounds today, it reminded me of the footage I've seen of concentration camp victims in WW II or from Bosnia in the mid-1990s.

6. More than usual, I noticed so many barefoot children walking the halls of the hospital today. In the emergency department, when treating explosive injuries in children, I don't think twice when they're without any footwear because they've been carried in by patients and I've assumed that they've lost their shoes in the blast. But today was the

first time since our arrival that I observed so many kids with improper or no footwear walking the unclean hospital floors and outdoor courtyard.

7. No matter where you go on planet Earth, there will always be people who will graffiti on a wall "so and so was here," even in Arabic, and Gaza is no different.

In the afternoon our team received the sudden notification that our exit date has been moved from October 1 to September 29th, which means that we will now be leaving Gaza in less than 80 hours. Although I'm excited to return home to my family, my initial reaction was to have a sinking feeling in my chest, as I now have to start saying goodbye to my friends, leaving them in a war that they can't escape, but I can. The next few days will be extremely heavy and emotional.

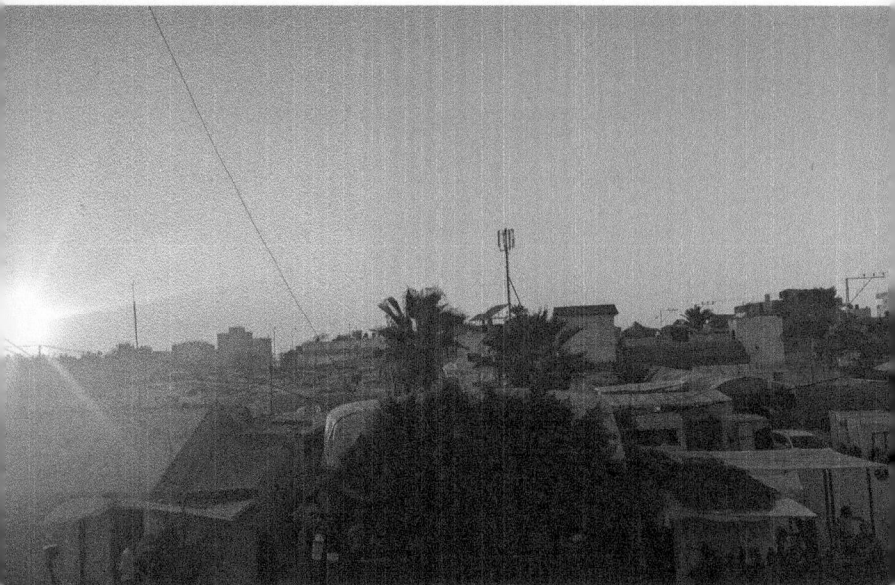

Sunset over Gaza from the ICU balcony at Al Aqsa Hospital

Day 27
September 26 – Why am I Here?

Why am I here? I don't mean it like "what the heck am I doing here?" But I'm asking myself the actual question of what was my intention and goal of coming to Gaza. I'm asking myself this question today because I want to renew my intentions and motivations to ensure I make the most of my last three days here, and don't simply count down the days until I return home, God Willing. The second reason is that it's a question that nearly everyone I've met has asked me.

The first reason is because of a dream I had several months ago that I've only shared with three people. Many would hear this and think, "You're crazy for making a life decision based on a dream." Although I do understand that dreams can reflect subconscious thoughts, I truly do believe there are dreams that can guide you if you're willing to listen to and trust them.

I think on some level, I still feel much guilt about not being able to do more to help the people here, undergoing what can only be described as hell on earth. I also wanted to see for my own eyes what is happening. Are the number of children and women being killed and maimed accurate? Are humanitarian zones *actually* being bombed?

I'm fortunate to be in a profession that is being allowed entry into Gaza, when it is inaccessible for most others. If you have any Palestinian ancestry, you cannot enter Gaza. This isn't a rumor but is asked as part of the WHO screening questions by every NGO; when the IDF and COGAT discover that you have a parent or grandparent who is Palestinian, they will refuse your entry into Gaza. It therefore falls to the rest of the world outside of Palestinians to help.

I'm under no delusion that my presence here is making a massive difference in clinical outcomes. The physicians and nurses here are masters at working in trauma under low resource settings. I know that whoever lived and died during my time here was going to live and die whether I was here or not. I am hopeful that my presence here allowed some of the doctors here a little respite when they needed a break or a second fresh brain.

I came here to be a witness, but I worry that my words and stories of the patients and families may not have the ability to change hearts like I thought they might. I still have to try though.

It's hard to explain, but I needed to be here to talk to them, see them, hug them, pat them on the back and say that I'm here just to be with them. Ultimately, you can probably say that I came here for me.

When talking with my friend Khalil, who is a second-year resident in orthopedic surgery, he reminded me that being here doesn't mean we have shared experiences. While I'm staying in the relative safety of the hospital at night, he goes home to a tent that could be bombed at any given moment. While my movements outside of the hospital are coordinated by the IDF, his are not. Why do I get the luxury of this protection and not him? I get the sense that he dislikes the idea that people think my life is in any real danger.

When I'm working, I can simply go across the street to buy whatever food I need with US$2800 that I brought into Gaza for one month. He is supporting his entire family on less than US$200 per month, and food insecurity is a real thing for him. I'm not worried about the safety and security of my family back home. While at work, he's constantly worrying about his family being bombed or attacked by thieves.

Talking to my other friend Khalil, the third-year ER resident, his wife is eight months pregnant with their first child, a boy who he plans to name Muhammad. They live in a tent about one kilometer from the hospital, and he has to make sure that he is home with her by 10 pm every night because it's not safe for her to be alone. He has no electricity so he has to charge his devices in the hospital. He has to walk 1.5 km each way to get water that lasts him two days. He used to be extremely muscular but now has lost a ton of weight. He told me once last week, "You know, I used to be a funny person and made jokes all the time." But now his mind is full of a hundred worries. He used to have textbooks memorized word for word but his mind has become clouded with "too many thoughts." Although we have worked together the past month in the same city and same hospital, I don't have even a fraction of his struggles and our lives just happen to be running in parallel for a time.

Back to orthopedic surgery Khalil again, I asked him what message he wanted me to take back to the West. His reply was: "You've had a year to help us and most of you haven't been willing to sacrifice even a little bit of your comfort to speak the truth. So don't worry about us; we have one test and that is to be patient. You have many tests that you have to overcome: greed, free time, and all of your privilege in the West that has caused you to be lazy about fighting for justice. Don't worry about us. Fix yourselves first."

He's 26 years old and he has lost several members of his immediate family. His career is on hold, and he's understandably angry and frustrated. He told me last week, "I've already grieved the future I'll never have." I know some of his anger is towards me and people like me, but I can't argue with him because it's not up to me to dictate how he responds to a crisis I did nothing to prevent. He didn't say any of this to be mean, but I asked him and he shared what was in his heart and I do believe that I needed to hear it to reflect on it for myself. His opinion, however, is in the minority of those that I've met. Most of the doctors and nurses are happy and feel touched that we left the comfort and security of our home to be with them during their hardship. My friend Anwar's mom woke up at 5 am to make us maftool last Friday and has sent *ma'mul* date cookies which she made with incredible love. When she met Israar she said there was "a light in Gaza now that you are here." These are nice things to hear and they make you feel good, but I think it's more important for me personally to take home what my orthopedics friend said, as it will motivate me more than the feeling of "I already did my part by coming here." In the end, all I could tell my friend Khalil is that I love him and then I promise to do better when I return home.

I can't pretend that I'm living a difficult life in my month here when my colleagues and friends have it exponentially harder. I also can't ignore or deny the fact that it's been 22 straight days of nearly daily carnage and chaos in the ER and my body is starting to wear down a little bit. But I have to remember that months ago, I would have given anything to spend even a day here, and have to use my remaining days wisely and ensure that I can give the staff the energy and focus they deserve to give them some relief.

If I've failed to live up to this, then I hope to still keep part of my promise by telling the world about them, in the hopes that it can move even a single person into action.

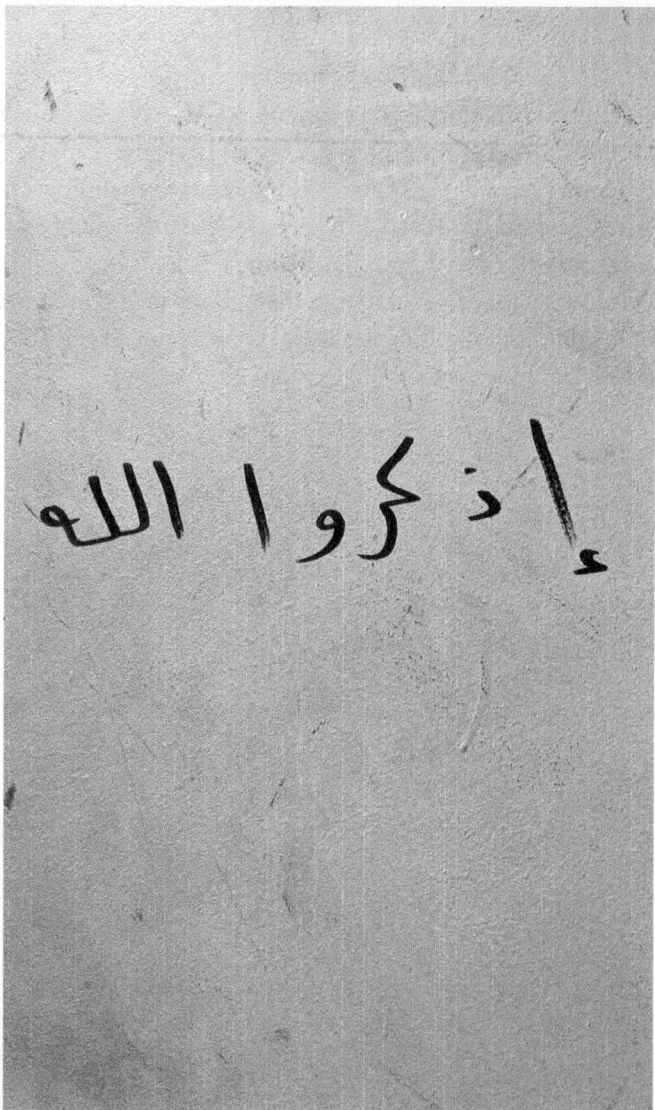

إ ذ كروا الله

Remember God, scrawled onto the wall of
a hallway in Al Aqsa Hospital

Day 28
September 27 – Forgotten

We went to sleep at 1:30 am last night, but not because it was busy. We spent the evening in the ER catching up with friends who we were seeing for the last time before our departure. We turned most of the lights off in the Red Zone so that the flies would go elsewhere and chatted in the dimly lit room for hours. We talked about philosophy, books (a lot about Dostoevsky's *Crime and Punishment*). We talked about the conflict and the dreaded October 7th, a date that I'm sure will be a day of mourning here in Gaza, as this was "the day they started killing all of us." No one I've spoken with remembers October 7 fondly. Instead, everyone remembers exactly where they were when they heard the news, and all of them instantly understood that their lives as they knew it were over. We talked about plans once the bombs stop. Many want to get married, and others want to resume their medical education. Some want to leave Gaza and start fresh elsewhere as they don't see a future here. We even listened to stories of those who were imprisoned and tortured for three to four months only to be set free with no explanation. At one point during a description of a horrible stress position torture technique, a nurse told the storyteller "Dr. Saleh, stop boring everyone and get to the interesting part." Even in a hospital across the world, the ER is the home of dark humor.

There were no critical patients so we talked late into the night until it was time to sleep. Once word had gotten around that we are scheduled to leave in two days, most of the ER team of physicians came by to wish us well. Nearly every physician and nurse asked us: "Will you return to Gaza?" or "You must return when there is peace and visit me when I rebuild my home."

At exactly 3 am, we were woken by the loudest explosion of the entire trip, one that shook not only the room, but the entire hospital. I woke up in a sweat and a bit of a panic for the first time with my heart racing and needed a moment to clear my head and figure out what exactly happened. An Apache helicopter fired a missile at a tent less than 100 ft away from the entrance of the ER, next to the courtyard where I often sit to get fresh air. One person was killed and three people were injured. These tents around the hospital are clearly part of the IDF designated safe/humanitarian zone. When my colleagues hear this term, they scoff because they know that nowhere in Gaza is truly safe.

I went online on September 24th, which was the worst day of our mission, and again last night to see if any of what I had witnessed was covered by any media. None of what I witnessed on September 24th was newsworthy. Even the violation of the humanitarian zone, where families have clustered for safety, wasn't even worth a mention. I like to believe that at other times, these would have been considered massacres that demanded the world's attention, but after one year, it's not even a footnote. It is clear to me now what wasn't clear to me a month ago: the world has forgotten about this place.

After our final Friday prayers in Gaza, our friend Anwar (who worked the night shift last night) brought us lunch, his mother's homemade maqluba. He found the ingredients on his way home from work and his mom prepared it for over four hours. It was the best meal I have ever eaten in my entire life, and was his family's parting gift to us.

Today we had planned to break with protocol and go to the beach in Deir Al Balah, which is only 1.5 km away, and you can easily see from the roof of the hospital. We hoped to spend a couple of hours by the water in the days before we departed for home. We were feeling a false sense of confidence because that area of the beach hadn't been bombed in quite some time. But this all changed at 11 pm the night before, when we received multiple casualties from the exact spot on the beach that we were planning on visiting. We took this as a sign that our day trip was not meant to be.

Dr. Fowzi and his 16-year-old son joined us for the meal as well and he also brought us gifts of a sweet date jam that he spent five hours preparing from his tent in Khan Yunis. We should be the ones who are giving these amazing people gifts, but their hearts are so big that they still feel honored and want to show us love. The generosity of the Ghazzawis is something I will never forget.

I had a long conversation with Dr. Fowzi after lunch, where we sat beside each other on the small foam mattress where I sleep. He took a deep sigh and said, "*Wallahi* [by God], I'm really going to miss you guys." I asked when he thinks peace will come and he lacked the optimism he displayed when we first met on September 3rd (if you remember our conversation). He sighed again and said, "I don't know when peace will come. Honestly we are so tired. The men are tired. The women are tired. The children are tired. This is hell."

We meet Dr. Fowzi about two to three times per week, and he's always making jokes, smiling and upbeat. But over the course of the month, his jubilant demeanor has slowly given way to a weariness. When I asked if he would ever leave, he replied, "How can we? We're trapped." He then paused and corrected himself "but we will never leave. This is our home. This is my parents' home, my grandfather's home. I'll stay until my death."

We continue to talk, he mentioned that his teenage kids are back in "school," which takes place in a tent run by volunteers that his kids dislike attending. They sit in the sand without chairs or desks, and most students don't have pen or paper. There is no blackboard so the students simply pay attention and try to remember what they can.

It is now 30 minutes past midnight. As I write this, several large explosions just went off, once again shaking our room. Just as I did on September 3, I'm imagining the terror and carnage currently taking place at wherever these bombs landed. The only difference between September 3 and today is that on September 3rd I thought the world was still watching, but today I know that no one is.

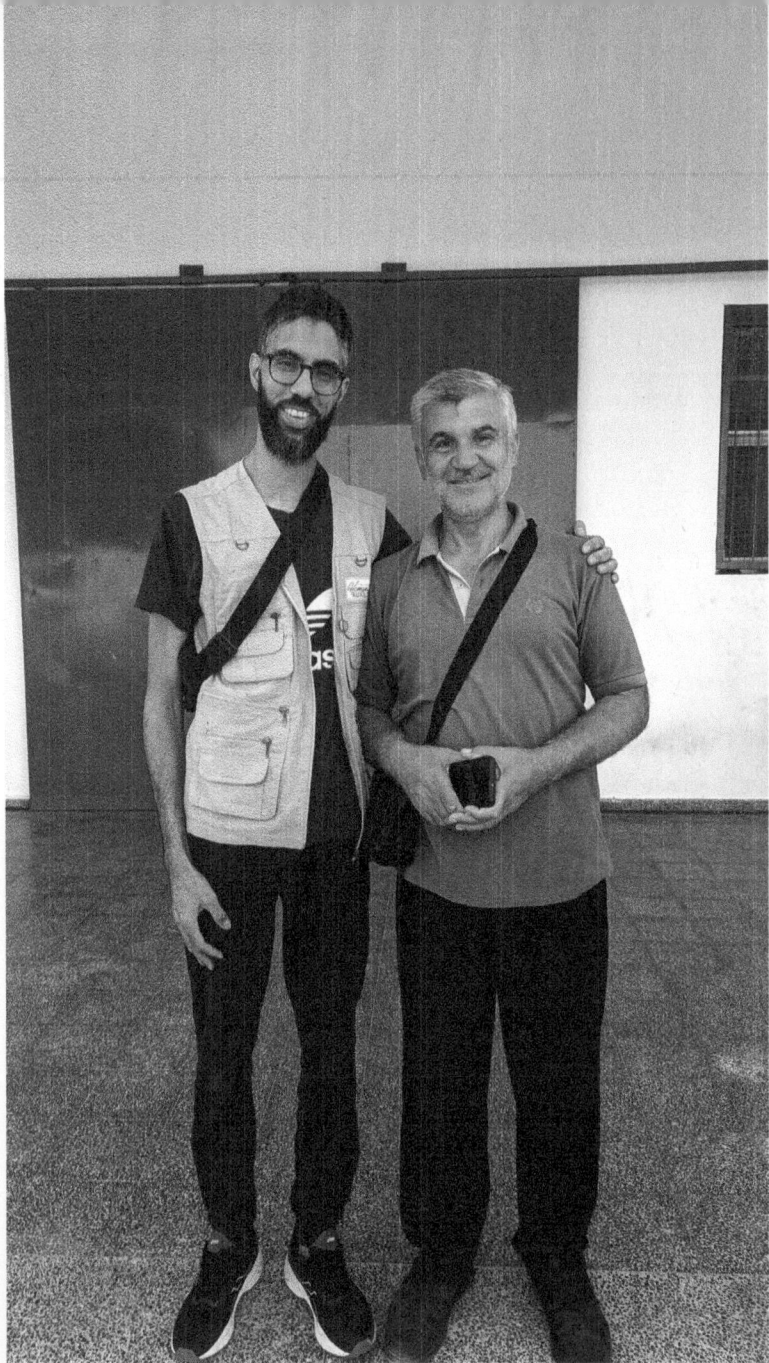

My friend Dr. Muhammad Al Aqqad (aka Dr. Fowzi)

Day 29
September 28 – Goodbyes

Today was one of the most emotional days I've ever experienced. It was a day that I've been nervous about for weeks. Today is my final day in Gaza. At times, it has felt like time stood still and at other times, I wondered how time could possibly move so fast. Despite the fact that I've had four weeks here, the past five days have seemed so abrupt.

We went down to the ER, not with the intention of working, but to say goodbye to our friends and colleagues working the day shift. Instead of having a moment like we did two nights ago, we arrived at a scene we have unfortunately become accustomed to greeting us every day—a mass casualty with absolute chaos in the ER, with the waiting room floor covered full of patients with "minor" injuries and the Red Zone full of critically injured patients. We put on our gloves for the final time in Gaza and tried to help as best as we could.

After about 90 minutes, the sickest three patients were stabilized and moved to the operating room. One had blood around his heart from a blast injury, preventing his heart from beating. The others suffered severe burns that made it look like they were placed in an incinerator with multiple shrapnel wounds piercing their pelvis. When the ER finally settled down, we now had the window to start saying goodbye to the friends we are leaving behind. This scene in the morning is the reason why leaving Gaza is weighing so heavily upon me today.

We spent some time in the office of the ER director Dr. Fahd Haddad and my friends Muhammad, Yahya and Mahmoud. Everyone keeps asking us "when will you come back to Gaza?" and my answer is always the same: "hopefully soon and in peace." But the reality is I don't know when I'm coming back. If there is a ceasefire soon, which is my hope, there will be no need for trauma ER doctors and the need will shift to family doctors, surgeons and other specialists. As much as I want to return in the next few months, for the sake of my friends, I hope I'm told very soon that my medical skills are no longer needed.

Leaving Gaza tomorrow is especially difficult for two reasons. The first is the guilt of me having the privilege of leaving when they are trapped. Simply because of my place of birth and the passport I hold, I get to leave to the safety and comfort of my family at home, which doesn't feel fair. In fact, it isn't fair. In the weeks leading up to my arrival, I was hoping and praying that a ceasefire would happen. These hopes only intensified once I began witnessing the daily carnage with my own eyes. Selfishly, I hoped to be here on that day to witness the outpouring of emotion that will take place in the hospital and on the streets. But this is selfish, as I haven't lost anyone or sacrificed anything to make that day about me. That day belongs to those who have lived this yearlong nightmare. I was hopeful that my departure would occur when there was peace, but seeing the mass casualties in the ER when I came to say goodbye was a reminder of how little has changed from our first to our last day here. Leaving my friends under these circumstances leaves me with a guilt that is impossible to shake.

The second reason leaving is so difficult, is because there is no relief from the constant bombs in Gaza. Even after one year, it is still one of the most dangerous places on Earth. There is the very real possibility that many of the people I've met will be dead before a permanent ceasefire occurs. "I will see you again" is more of a wish than an actual promise I can keep.

After saying farewell to the daytime ER staff, we returned to our room where Dr. Fowzi brought us a homemade lunch of delicious rice and chicken. It took him nearly three hours and two taxis to bring this to the Al Aqsa Hospital from his tent in Khan Yunis. It was also flattering that several of our friends who weren't even scheduled to work today visited us on their day off to say farewell.

The first was our ER friend Anwar, who brought us gifts from his mom to my wife and daughters: a beautiful hand embroidered purse, and two traditional red Palestinian shawls for them. To think that after all he has done for me to welcome me here and make me feel a part of his family, he still brought gifts for my family that he has never met. I am at a loss for words to describe this generosity and selflessness. Despite living in a tent for the past year the love they have shown me is something that I'm still trying to comprehend. When it was finally time to part ways, I walked him to the hospital gates, hugged my dear friend knowing that there's a very real possibility that I will never see him again. We promised to stay in touch and that we would meet again. And then just like that, he turned his back, walked to the street and disappeared into the night and an uncertain future.

After lunch, Dr. Fowzi fell asleep on my mattress in a post-food coma. When he woke up, he shared that he hasn't slept that comfortably in nearly one year, saying that his tent is "too uncomfortable," and he hasn't fallen asleep inside the safety and comfort of an actual building in so long. When it was time to leave, it was hard to say goodbye. He told us that he lost his brother in a bombing seven months ago, and that Israar and I are his new brothers. "I'm certain we will meet again, either in this life or the next." The last people to visit us was our ER friend Khalil (who is expecting a son any day now) and Abu Musa, who works in IT at the hospital, and who we spend time with every few days. After an hour, filled with the usual "butterflies in your stomach" feeling of knowing you have to say goodbye, we once again hugged each other and promised that we would see each other again, but not really knowing for sure.

We met Abu Musa in our favorite spot in the hospital, on the ICU balcony overlooking the ER steps and court-yard of the Al Aqsa Hospital, where we've enjoyed watching the children play below while soaking in the evening breeze for the final time. Earlier today, Abu Musa gifted me with a Palestinian kefiyyeh, which is a distinctly patterned black and white scarf that he wrapped around my neck while saying "Now, you are an official Ghazzawi."

My final goodbye was reserved for someone who hasn't spoken a word to me, but still managed to steal my heart. I'm referring to four-year-old Yusuf, my beautiful friend who has been in the ICU since his head and lung injuries on September 10. He was awake when I saw him, just staring at me, appearing frightened and jittery, likely as a reaction to the explosion and also a three-week ICU stay. He is slowly on the mend, but will require help with mechanical ventilation through his tracheostomy for some time, until he gets the strength to be weaned off it. I will probably never see Yusuf again, and he has likely already forgotten me, but I will remember him for the rest of my life. He reminds me so much of my four-year-old son, and I already miss him.

Today has weighed heavily on my heart. The act of saying goodbye to someone, potentially forever, is difficult but necessary. I've written about the importance of families needing closure for their dying family members, and saying goodbye to a friend you may never see again is equally important. If I measure my impact in Gaza purely by clinical outcomes, then what I contributed in my four weeks here wasn't enough. But if you include the relationships made and the friendships formed, only then can I maybe hope to justify my presence. And that is why saying goodbye to my friends was so important, allowing me to close one of the most important chapters in the story of my life.

This place is full of people who have entered my life and now left it like a flash of lightning. I needed them to know that they had a greater impact on my life than I had on theirs. I needed them to know that despite our short time together, I love them and they will always be with me. But on some level, I think I also needed to know that they felt the same way, and that there was more in their eyes than my own reflection staring back at me, and that I mattered to them too. When I parted with many of my friends, they would say the famous line: *Wa Antum Minna wa Nahnu Minkum*, which means "You are of us, and we are of you" and is one of the greatest honors of my life. The memory of these moments will stay with me for as long as I live.

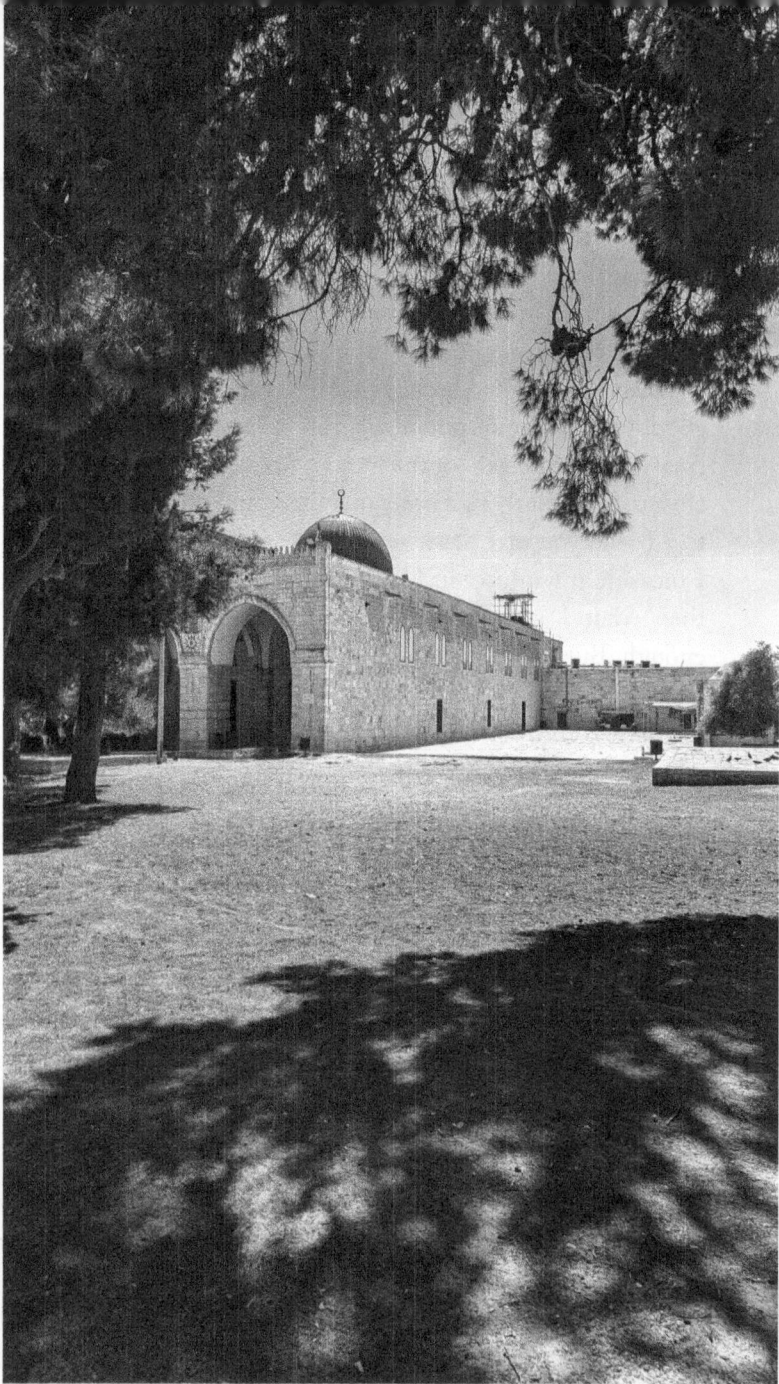

Masjid Al Aqsa, the 3rd holiest site in Islam

Day 31
September 30 – Final Reflections

I'm starting this final post from the comfort of my hotel room overlooking downtown Amman. Less than two days ago, I was living a minimalist existence inside of Gaza, and now I'm surrounded by incredible luxury. Tonight, I will sleep in a hotel room, while my friends and colleagues left behind will be sleeping in tents in a displacement camp. I have refrained from using the word "refugee" because they are proud and accomplished people who plan on returning to and rebuilding their homes when it is safe and whenever that day comes. It will still take weeks to process my experience over this past month, and I'm sure my perspective will take time to form, but nonetheless, I still wanted to share my final thoughts before signing off on this journal.

My intention behind writing was to shine a light on the people of Gaza and to bring their struggles and stories to the front and center of the consciousness of my circle of friends. I am blessed to have many people who care about me and will be curious as to how I'm doing, so I'll address it here. I felt a wide range of emotions including grief, anger, anxiety, sadness, frustration and guilt. I've wept on many occasions while in Gaza, and often while writing these entries, and speaking about them will transport me back to the moment they happened. I've seen innocent adults and children suffer gruesome deformities and heard their screams of fear and pain as well as from their families. I will undoubtedly have moments where the memory of these sights, sounds and smells will become fresh again, causing me to struggle to finish sentences when speaking about them. But I'm confident that in time, I'll be able to channel these emotions into productive work and advocacy, God willing.

I am blessed to have an unshakable faith which constantly reminds me that behind everything that happens, big and small, good and evil, there is a wisdom that is veiled from me which is beyond my comprehension. This doesn't mean that we simply sit back and allow injustice to occur. Rather, it is this belief that allows me to stay motivated even when I don't see the results with my own eyes. Without this faith in The Creator, I would go absolutely mad.

The carnage, terror and injustice I have witnessed has undoubtedly changed me. I am not the same person that I was on September 2. As the days and weeks passed, I could feel my heart and mind changing into a different version of myself. After what I have seen, how could I possibly remain unchanged? My spiritual belief has been reaffirmed and even strengthened in many ways. However, many of the Western values that I have come to believe in throughout the course of my life, I now understand to be hollow. I still don't know exactly who this new Salman will be, but there are changes that I must make in my life in order for my time in Gaza to be truly transformative and have meaning. It is impossible to view the world with the same eyes as before I left.

I'll be departing for home in six hours and I can't wait to hold my family. Nearly every child I've treated here has reminded me of my own kids in some manner. Even the privilege of being excited to see my wife and children at the airport is not lost on me and is something that many of my friends and colleagues in Gaza do not have. My four weeks in Gaza have heightened my awareness of the incredible privilege I possess. It is very clear to me that where I am in life has nothing to do with how hard I have worked or any sacrifice I've made, and is almost exclusively determined by the location of my birth and who my parents are—two factors I had no control over. I've worked alongside doctors and nurses who possess more knowledge and who have worked harder than me, yet here I stand. I am not saying privilege is a bad thing or something that we have to hide—quite the opposite. I think it's important to wield our privilege, not to simply bring ease, comfort or happiness to our own lives, but to create a more just world for those who lack what we have. To speak against injustice without fear and to use our resources to move people. If we can't do this, it feels like our privilege is a wasted blessing.

Today I was able to fulfill a lifelong dream and visit Masjid Al Aqsa in Jerusalem, the third most important site in Islam. This was a trip that seemed impossible only one week ago and I was specifically instructed to remove this idea from my brain before I departed in August. I let go of the idea until about ten days ago when Israar asked if I thought it was possible. I have an incredible story to share about the power of a prayer called "*Istikhara*," so remind me to share this with you when we meet. Once again, my immense privilege was made apparent to me. I turned 42 while in Gaza and if me, my parents or grandparents were born in Palestine, I would not be allowed to enter Masjid Al Aqsa. There were multiple IDF soldiers and police guarding every entrance of the mosque as well as everywhere in the courtyard. I have been told that the Israeli police do not allow Palestinian men under the age of 55 to enter and pray at Al Aqsa. This statement alone should be enough to demonstrate the weight of the oppressive occupation experienced by the Palestinians. Once we arrived at the gates, we were met by IDF soldiers and police carrying large automatic assault rifles, ready to turn us away. But once we flashed our UK and Canadian passports, abracadabra, we were allowed to enter a place that we would be unable to if we were Palestinian. I felt incredibly fortunate to walk the streets of the Old City, and to walk the grounds of the Noble Sanctuary. It felt like I was given a gift to visit Al Aqsa, and was the closure I needed before retuning home.

What about the Palestinians? What type of closure do they receive? They are still being killed in Gaza on a daily basis by indiscriminate bombings, quadcopters, and Apache helicopters with an average death toll ranging from 15 to 70 per day. The reason I felt compelled to go to Gaza is that despite the lack of media attention and eyes shifting elsewhere in the region, Gaza remains the most important news story on planet Earth today.

I have no Palestinian blood coursing through my veins and my parents' land of origin, Pakistan, has its own ongoing internal crises of human rights. What the Palestinians in both the West Bank and especially Gaza are going through resonates with me because I believe it is a litmus test for all of us who live in the West. Do we really stand for human rights for all people, or only a select few? How can we claim to champion women's rights without standing for the women giving birth in the streets and menstruating without health products? Do we really believe in protecting children when I've now witnessed an entire generation of children being maimed, killed, orphaned and amputated? Are we all willing to accept the psychologic trauma experienced by children who are being bombed without warning or explanation, with the people they trust the most being unable to protect them? If we don't act now, are we all okay with *another* 25,000 women and children being killed? Have we all accepted the term "collateral damage" as a humane way to rationalize the carnage inflicted on the most vulnerable?

I ask these questions to all of us rather than asking of the many other humanitarian crises across our planet because our institutions of power, leadership and finance are complicit in creating the current conditions in Gaza. Our governments in Canada, the United States and the United Kingdom are still providing both financial support in the form of weapons and political cover for the daily killings of children in Gaza. Our banks and institutions of higher learning are invested heavily in weapons manufacturers that are supplying the arms that are murdering innocent humans and civilians. Our major corporations have invested heavily in companies that are funding oppression in the occupied Palestinian territories and facilitating what many major global human rights organizations (including Israeli ones) and the International Court of Justice have labeled an apartheid system against the Palestinian people.

When saying goodbye to my friends and colleagues, none of them asked me to tell the world about them because I share a religion and many similar values and they knew I would share their message. When Victoria (who is a Caucasian female American physician from New York) said goodbye, they felt the need to ask her: "Please tell the people in your country that we are good people who love peace." This broke my heart. After an entire year of being massacred and forcibly evicted from their homes, they believe that this is happening because people in the West think they are bad people who deserve this in some way, because they are savages who love death. This narrative sounds so familiar to anyone who has read a history book.

As beautiful as the Palestinians of Gaza are, they are not perfect. After one year of this chaos, the social fabric of the society is falling apart. There is a palpable air of incredible desperation in every corner of society that has left no one untouched. What they want all of us to know is that they are not okay and they are in desperate need of our help. Here are the ways that I believe anyone reading this can help:

1. Do not be afraid to speak about Gaza. I had heard from colleagues over the past year who have told me, "you can't talk about that" or "you're going to get into trouble" or "you're making people feel uncomfortable." As long as your speech isn't hateful and you are positively promoting Palestinian rights, keep advocating. I'm not asking you to risk your career or livelihood, but if speaking for a ceasefire in Gaza and for Palestinian human rights places your job and your career in jeopardy, maybe we're operating in a system worth opposing that we should all be fighting to change.

2. Be mindful of the products you buy and where your money is going. You would be surprised to learn how many of our products are from companies whose parent corporations are heavily invested in weapons manufacturers, or invested in companies operating in illegal settlements in

the occupied West Bank. If you can find affordable alternatives, boycott these products. When speaking to people in Gaza, they truly value the solidarity of boycotting products contributing to their oppression. It may not bankrupt these companies, but even if it offers Palestinians a glimmer of hope, it's a worthwhile endeavor.

3. Write letters and sign petitions to your elected officials, financial institutions and universities that you are alumni of, demanding them to divest immediately from any weapons manufacturers and corporations which are invested in enabling the killing of civilians in Gaza.

4. Read and keep yourself informed to keep Gaza in the forefront of our collective consciousness. After one year, it is no longer an acceptable or charming excuse to say this issue is "too complicated."

5. Donate. From what I've learned on the ground, US$2000 can currently feed a family of five in Gaza for an entire year. There is a scarcity of vital supplies and food in Gaza, and liquidity of cash is low. There are multiple avenues to have funds reach directly into the hands of those who need it inside Gaza.

My plane is about to board shortly, and I am bursting with excitement at the thought of seeing and holding my family again. I'll take a few days to rest and enjoy family time, but then my work to keep the promises I made to my friends begins.

God Willing:

I will keep advocating for the people of Gaza, and my friends and colleagues. I will never shy away from speaking up against the killing of civilian men, women and children.

I will return to this land, and I will return with my wife and children to help rebuild.

I will return to see my friends: Anwar, Khalil, Fahd, Walid, Yahya, Mahmoud, Abdallah, Abu Musa, Shahdi, Israa, Donya, Saleh, Amr, Muhamad Al Aqqad (Dr. Fowzi), and everyone who has forever changed my life. I will eat meals of maqluba, maftool and musakhan in their homes.

I will hug them and weep, and beg them for forgiveness for failing to do more to prevent what has happened to them.

Until my last breath, I will not stop using my voice for Palestine.

Alhamdulillah, all praise is due to The Most High for bringing me to this land and honoring me with serving the people of Gaza at this time in history. My month in Gaza has been and will likely remain as the greatest honor of my life, outweighing my medical degree or any title I've held. By every objective metric, Gaza is one of the worst places on Earth. Yet, my heart has never been more still than in the four weeks I've spent here. I don't know what good I have done in my life to deserve this honor, but I will forever be grateful for it.

* * *

I would like to thank the founder of Humanity Auxilium, Dr. Fozia Alvi for trusting me with this massive responsibility. I also would like to thank the director of operations, Dr. Faiza Hussain for providing our team with the preparation, tools and resources to perform our work to the best of our abilities. Dr. Hussain facilitated every aspect of our medical mission and without her, our work in Gaza would have been impossible. Thank you to Israar and Victoria for their friendship during our month away from home.

Most importantly, thank you to my beloved wife Areej, who without her encouragement and support, my journey and work would be impossible. As an ER physician herself, I know that her heart wishes she was in Gaza with me. I pray that the sacrifice she made to stay home and take care of our children will be rewarded just the same. To have a spouse who knows what you're feeling and encourages you to act on a dream is one of life's greatest joys and I will never take her companionship for granted.

Lastly, thank you to all of you for reading my journal and daily reflections. I have opened up my heart in a way that I never have before in the hopes that you or someone that you know might be moved into helping to end the suffering of the people of Gaza. Thank you for all of your words of encouragement and support.

I pray that God accepts my intentions and my actions. Anything good I have done is from Him, The Most High, and only the mistakes belong to me.

With love and respect,

Your friend and brother, Salman

Then he came back.

Left side: The last page of my diary entry; Right side:
My six-year-old daughter's contribution to the diary

Afterword

Diana Buttu

As I write, a "ceasefire" has just been announced by the Qatari Foreign Minister. The ceasefire will involve the end of Israel's brutal attacks on Gaza and the release of Palestinian prisoners and hostages, for the release of the Israelis who continue to be held in Gaza. Palestinians around the world rejoiced, finally feeling that the Israel's genocide is now coming to an end.*

While Israeli bombs may no longer be dropping, the wholesale devastation that Israel wrought on Palestinians is just beginning to be felt. Palestinians are returning to their cities—now in complete ruins. In some cases, they are digging out their loved ones from beneath the rubble, hoping to provide a dignified burial to those who did not survive Israeli bullets and bombs. People are turning to social media to ask for information about those who were killed; seeking specifics like where they were buried so that they can visit their graves. Others are posting pictures of friends and family who are missing and presumed to be held in Israeli torture camps like Sde Teiman where thousands of people from Gaza are being held.

For the thousands of Palestinians who are from the north—places like Beit Hanoun and Jabaliya—they are returning to find only rubble. The images are apocalyp-

---

* Israel violated the ceasefire within eight weeks.

tic, leaving me imagining the level of hate that Israelis have towards Palestinians to inflict this much damage to homes, schools, gardens, and so on. One of Israel's ministers, Bezalel Smotrich, assured Israelis that "Gaza is destroyed and broken, uninhabitable, and it will remain so." In some places, not a single structure remains intact. It is estimated that Israel has destroyed more than 88 percent of Palestinian homes and buildings in Gaza. Israeli bombs targeted every university and the majority of schools and many shelters. Basic infrastructure, such as telecommunications, sewage, water, and electricity, were not spared.

But Israel inflicted the greatest damage to the health sector—deliberately—in order to ensure that Palestinian life cannot resume, for without healthcare, survival is difficult. This is why Israel began its slick *hasbara* campaign, including video animations, aimed at justifying its attack on the healthcare system. Some journalists happily and whole-heartedly parroted Israeli talking points, paving the way for these illegal bombings. One does not need to be an expert in international law to know that targeting hospitals is illegal. Yet, over the course of 15 months, the Israeli army bombed virtually all of the hospitals leaving only half of the hospitals partially (not fully) functioning. Israel killed 950 medical workers, including doctors, nurses, and paramedics, and continues to hold 200 hostages in secret prisons.

It is in this context that Dr. Salman Khalid's work in Gaza must be understood. He beautifully highlights what it was like to be living and working in Gaza during the genocide and the desperate but valiant efforts to try to treat and help as many people as possible, under a collapsed health care system. He describes in a way that we can only imagine the types of injuries that he saw and treated, due to the different types of weapons tested out on Palestinians. As we watched the endless TikToks of Israeli soldiers proudly displaying their sadism, Dr. Khalid and his colleagues were on the receiving end. He and his colleagues brought humanity, tenderness and love to people who have been so deprived of human kindness due to Israeli and American policies. In his journal, Dr. Khalid also manages to bring forth the generosity and gentle spirit of the people of Gaza whom the world has forsaken and ignored, preferring instead to side with a nuclear power (Israel) over a stateless, refugee (overwhelmingly child) population.

But what strikes me most about Dr. Khalid's journal is when he asks himself what he is doing in Gaza. Yes, he treated many, many individuals—for which I and others are so thankful—and in the process realizes that his work is not simply that of a physician, but of a person who has come to give (and receive) love. It is impossible to leave Gaza without a sense that the people deserve so much more. It is impossible to leave Gaza without feeling loved. Simply put, solidarity is mutual love. And it is that mutual love that Israel will never feel. Israel will never know what it is like for people around the world to stand in solidarity with it. It will never see global protests in support. Israel will never have student encampments in support. Rather, Israel will only ever see global efforts to boycott and ostracize it and to hold Israeli war criminals to account—deservedly so—for war criminals are not loved around the world.

Dr. Khalid asks why he was in Gaza. It was to give and receive love. And with this book, he has guided you to do the same. The mutual love that Dr. Khalid experienced is so deeply rooted that it is unstoppable despite Israeli efforts to crush it. It is a love that is so strong that it will catapult us— all of us—to a freedom we all deserve.

Diana Buttu
January 2025

The Pluto Press Newsletter

Hello friend of Pluto!

Want to stay on top of the best radical books
we publish?

Then sign up to be the first to hear about our
new books, as well as special events,
podcasts and videos.

You'll also get 50% off your first order with us
when you sign up.

Come and join us!

Go to bit.ly/PlutoNewsletter